Robert Spindl

CW01500241

My Oldtime Strongman Training

How to Build Old School Strength and Muscle, Master
Classic Feats of Strength, and Perform Them

Published by the Author
Innsbruck 2020

Disclaimer

The information in this book is to be used at your own risk and is no replacement for professional health care advice. The author strongly advises you to consult a physician prior to beginning a physical training program. If you experience any discomfort or pain performing the exercises described in this book or following the advice given in it, interrupt your training immediately and seek qualified advice.

For reasons of readability and history, the masculine form is used throughout this book. All information applies to all genders.

First edition

© Robert Spindler
Published by the Author
Innsbruck 2020

www.eisen-hans.at

ISBN: 9798654211651

To my brother Richard

Table of contents

1. Introduction: The legacy of the German oldtime strongmen

Although I grew up in, and still live in, the mountainous Austrian Tyrol, and although I was born in German Bavaria – home of the oldtime strongman Hans Steyrer (1849-1906; famous for routinely lifting a 500 pound stone with only one finger) – my family roots lie in a true hub of classic strength athletics. From both my mother's and father's side, my ancestors come from Eastern Germany, more precisely from Saxony, Thuringia, and Berlin.

Already back in the eighteenth century, Saxony had a legendary electoral prince, Friedrich August I. von Sachsen (1670-1733), commonly called *August der Starke* (Augustus the Strong), who broke horseshoes and rolled up silver plates in front of his distinguished guests, but also in front of his people, to win their sympathy.

In Leipzig, one of the major cities in Saxony, the famous Arthur Saxon (1878-1921) trained for his still unbeaten 168kg (371lbs) one-arm bent-press in 1905, in what I call the golden age of the strongmen. Leipzig is also where Hermann Görner (1891-1956) performed his legendary one-hand deadlift of 330kg (728lbs) in 1920. In Thuringia, people from the street today still remember Milo Barus (1906-1977), a Strongest Man of the World from 1930. In Berlin, the Jewish athlete Siegmund Breitbart (1893-1925) aka *Eisenkönig* (Iron King) bent horseshoes, broke chains, and eventually drove the fatal iron spike through a wooden board and accidentally into his thigh, which caused the blood poisoning that led to his tragic early death in 1925.

This golden age of the strongmen, the turn from the nineteenth to the twentieth century, must have been an interesting time. The French call it the *"Belle Époque"*, the "beautiful era", and the British still think ardently of their "Victorian" and "Edwardian" Ages. This period, the *"Wilhelminische Zeitalter"*, as it is known in Germany, was an era of economic thrive, revolutionary inventions, and successful foundings of companies – an optimistic age of improving hygienic conditions, revolutions in medicine, colourful world fairs, and spectacular entertainment, including the grandiose circuses, which we associate with the great strength athletes of the time. However, a lot of this optimism was superficial. The perceived luxury and flamboyance had went hand in hand with a growing divide between the very rich and a well-to-do middle class on the one side, and an exploited labour class on the other. Eventually, the powder keg exploded with the advent and terrible consequences of World War I. The war meant a great damper to the optimistic spirit in Europe and revealed that the era was not so great in retrospect. Thus, of all the different international denominations, Mark Twain's ironic "The Gilded Age" seems to be the most fitting term for the period.

Nevertheless, strongmen continued to thrive for another two decades after World War I, and many great athletes and feats of strength from these interbellum years are still remembered today. With the advent of World War II, however, the age of the classic strongmen ended once and for all. The Nazis had already experimented with performance-enhancing drugs, and in the ensuing cold war, Russians and Americans eventually drove similar experiments to perfection. Instead of the all-round strongmen of the pre-war years, strength sports now became more and more specialized. Eventually, it split clearly into bodybuilding, Olympic weightlifting, powerlifting, and, later on, the modern strongman sport. With few exceptions, great strength athletes now became either the one or the other, or they became wrestlers, shot putters, etc.

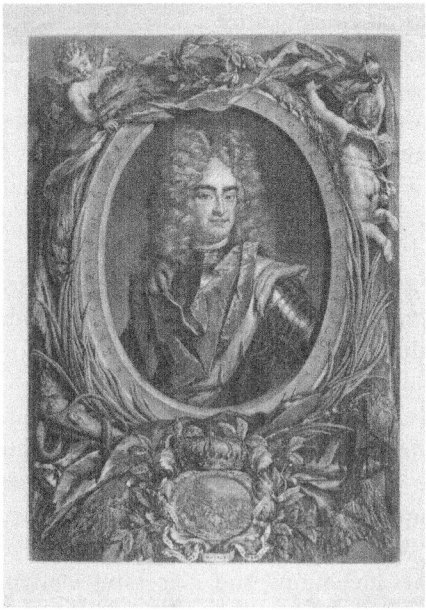

Figure 1.1 Friedrich August "*der Starke*" I. von Sachsen.

In the seventies, the first Strongest Man competitions still brought together athletes from a variety of these fields for a colourful, farcical media sensation. Later, the modern strongman sport became a very specialized discipline in its own right as well.

Thus, ever after World War II, strength sports were all about specialization and top performance in a narrow field, under the strict supervision of coaches, doctors, and sponsors. Systematically, strength sports became political, and it became impossible to achieve greatness without the support of a large, and often dubious, team of experts behind your back. Until the downfall of the Berlin Wall in 1989, Eastern Germany partly lived up to its reputation as a cradle of strength, but, as became public later on, this fame relied to a large degree on an efficient, institutionalized doping system.

Thus, the classical German strongmen had become a further indirect victim of World War II and the Nazi-regime, just like the ingenious German comedian Karl Valentin (1882-1948), the German Charlie Chaplin, as he was also called. The rejection of this German icon by the Nazis, and his tragic end in hunger and poverty, stand emblematic for how the fun and team spirit in strength sports must also have gradually vanished, and made place for, first, the malnutrition and deprivation of the war, and then the narcissism and systematic exploitation of individuals for political prestigious goals, and commercial endeavours, in the second half of the twentieth century.

Hermann Görner died poor and all but forgotten in 1956, and some will forever eye his old photographs with suspicion for his dubious moustache. The outspoken social democrat Milo Barus had survived interrogations through the Nazi Gestapo and five years' incarceration from 1936 to 1941, followed by forced labour in a quarry, until the end of the war. But apparently, his spirit could not be broken. After World War II, he took up his training again and continued to perform feats of strength in front of enthusiastic audiences, bringing excitement into the everyday lives of GDR (German Democratic Republic) citizens under the socialist regime. Until 1963, up to the age of 57, Barus tingled East-German villages to perform feats of strength for a few Pfennig or Deutsche Mark. The collective gratitude of the Thuringians for his eagerness is reflected in the fact that his memory is still kept alive with a little museum, in the secluded, green Thuringian valley where Barus had maintained a small restaurant, and a strongman competition that takes place there every year. However, outside of Thuringia the extent of Milo Baurs' fame is nowhere near where it is in his (temporary) chosen home country.

With Milo Barus, the positive role model of a natural, down-to-earth, neighbourhood strongman-type, who performs feats of strength before a crowd to make a living, practically died out. It made place for the colourful, flamboyant, and exaggerated worlds and bodies of modern bodybuilding and strength sports. Only very few men (and women) have kept the tradition of the performing oldtime strongman alive to this day. And only relatively recently has a niche in strength sports evolved out of the classic feats of strength. In our days, there exists a growing, worldwide community of grip strength-, steel bending-, stonelifting-, etc. enthusiasts. Slowly but surely, they are securing themselves a firm place in the convoluted universe of modern strength sports and physical culture.

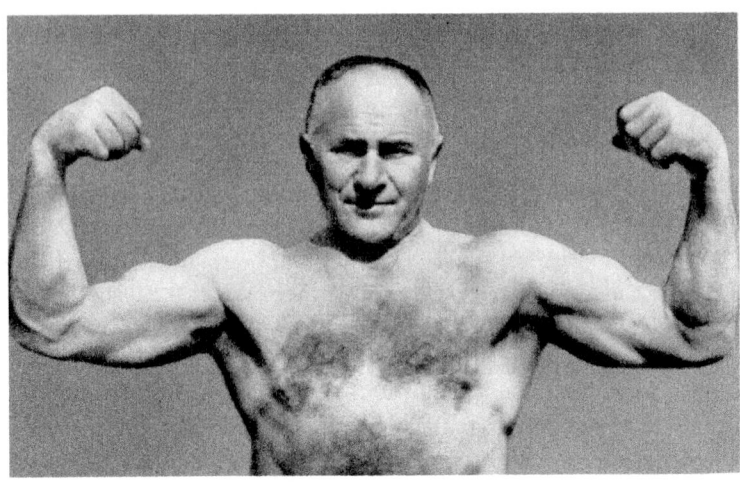

Figure 1.2 Milo Barus.

This book is for those interested in exactly this subculture of strength athletics, but also for those interested in the art of classic strongman performances, as well as in the history of strength sports. It comes from someone who does not claim to be the strongest or best in any particular discipline, but from someone who has managed, over many years of training, to achieve a diverse number of respectable benchmarks in various strength disciplines, naturally and mostly on his own, and, most notably, someone who has made a living out of performing feats of strength in front of many different audiences for more than ten years. The primary purpose of this book is to entertain, but I hope you will also find some information in it to serve your purposes, whatever they might be.

Innsbruck, July 2020

2. My definition of the oldtime strongman and oldtime strength

If the golden age of the (oldtime) strongmen is long past, what do I mean when I talk about oldtime strongman training in this book? The way I see it, Milo Barus was probably one of the last true oldtime strongmen, because his active career had started early and he simply continued his art after the war until he was already a kind of a relict, a living fossil. But World War II had been the decisive break of the twentieth century. Just as the world was not the same after this terrible event in many ways, the strength world was also not the same, as I have tried to show in my introductory chapter. All the other notable strong men and women who came after World War II, with the exception of people like Milo Barus, did something else than him and his predecessors. There are only very few exceptions of individuals who truly and honestly aspired, and continue to aspire, to the ideal of the oldtime strongman. This ideal – by my own and not binding definition is the following:

1. An oldtime strongman is an idealist. He strives towards the greatest attainable strength, without cheating, or short cuts. He despises fake feats of strength and he despises the use of substances to increase his potential at the risk of his own health, and at the risk of being a bad example to young admirers. He uses his strength only for the good, not against those weaker or less powerful, or to project arrogance or aggressiveness. He is honest and would not publicize manipulated films or photographs of himself to make the wrong impression of him having achieved a certain feat, or a level of physical development that he has, in actuality, not.

2. An oldtime strongman is a traditionalist and nostalgic. He disregards recent trends and developments in the strength world. He ignores the hype around novel training techniques, food supplements, and weightlifting equipment, and he is immune to the dictation of the world of fashion. Instead, he loves rusty barbells and tattered weightlifting booklets by Lionel Strongfort and Charles Atlas. An oldtime strongman steadfastly believes in the efficiency of simple and basic training methods and equipment, in the unalterable laws of physics, biology, leverage, gravity, and muscle growth. He studies training methods more than a hundred years old, and believes they are all that one needs to develop strength beyond the ordinary.

Thus:

3. An oldtime strongman is a minimalist. He believes that if he only had one form of resistance, only one tool to train his strength, be it a large stone, a steel bar, a heavy barbell, a piece of rope, wood, or chain, he would continue to develop and work on his strength until it reached a herculean level. He knows that progressive resistance, the continuing increase of weight, thickness of steel, or size of stone, combined with patience and perseverance, is the only thing that makes him stronger over time – not a fancy workout plan, exotic exercises, novel equipment, a recent diet, or the number of photographs he publicizes of himself while working out or flexing his muscles. All an oldtime strongman needs is a simple, straightforward workout plan. He knows that it is not the complexity of a training regimen that makes his muscles grow, but lots of time and hard work.

But:

4. An oldtime strongman is a universalist. Since an oldtime strongman stubbornly denies progress, he resists the trend towards further specialization, which surfaces in the strength world as in does in any other field, be it academia, business, or trade. An oldtime strongman might be an expert in a particular feat of strength, but he will make sure that he has an acceptable level of overall physical strength. He will also continue to work on other feats, even if he might not achieve a competitive level in those. An oldtime strongman will be aware that once he is commonly known as a strong man, he will have to face all sorts of challenges common people associate with strength. An oldtime strongman will be prepared for requests to do a certain number of push-ups or pull-ups, to lift some heavy person from the floor, to hoist several children into the air, to help move a particularly weighty piece of furniture, to move a heavy boulder, to open a stubborn jar of marmalade, or to bend some rusty horseshoe found in a riding stable.

Even if he might not be able to meet a certain challenge, he will partake in it with a smile and, if necessary, generously grant another the victory in some specialized feat in which that person takes great pride. An oldtime strongman will thus go a much longer way before the words "this is not my field" cross his lips, and before he raises his hand in denial (Perhaps the only exception being, by my advice, a challenge to an armwrestling match. This can not only lead to a surprising and shameful defeat, but also to injuries that can seriously disrupt a prospective strongman career). Some oldtime strongmen might also want to fulfil visual expectations to a strong man, like wide shoulders, a V-shaped back, a bulging biceps, and Herculean thighs, although it is common knowledge that a strong body and a strong-*looking* body are not necessarily the same. It might also be a wise move for an oldtime strongman to be prepared to meet play- or spiteful challenges to feats *not* commonly associated with a strong man, perhaps intended to reveal one's limitations, like a feat of endurance. In this regard, I am fully in line with the legendary Arthur Saxon, who said, as early as 1906:

> "The usual idea about strength – I mean the idea of the average reader of health magazines – is generally a wrong one. Although a weight-lifter […], I hope that I, personally, am broad-minded enough to recognise that a man does not prove himself an all-round strong man just because he is able to lift a heavy weight, especially when the weight is lifted once only. The following is my diagnosis of real strength:
>
> Genuine strength should include not only momentary strength, as proved by the ability to lift a heavy weight once, but also the far more valuable kind of strength known as strength for endurance. This means the ability, if you are a cyclist, to jump on your machine and ride 100 miles at any time without undue fatigue; if a wrestler, to wrestle a hard bout for half an hour with a good man without a rest, yet without becoming exhausted and reaching the limit of your strength.
>
> Apart from sports, enduring strength means that the business man shall stand, without a break-down, business cares and worries, that he shall be capable, when necessary, of working morning, afternoon and night with unflagging energy, holding tightly in his grasp he reins of business, retaining all the while a clear mind and untiring energy, both of body and brain. The man who can miss a night's rest or miss a meal or two without showing any ill effect or without losing any physical power, is better entitled to be considered a strong man than the man who is only apparently strong, being possessed of momentary strength, which is, after all, a muscle test pure and simple. In the latter case, where a man raises, once only, a heavy weight, all that he proves himself to possess is muscular control and great contractile power, but this does not guarantee sound internal organs, nor does it prove that a man would come out well in an endurance test. The man capable of long feats of endurance should live longest, and such a man will find his powers of more avail in everyday life than the man who has sacrificed vital strength for an extra few eighths of an inch of

muscle, and perhaps the ability to raise a few pounds more in a certain position in a weight-lifting test." (Saxon 23-24)

I could not agree more. And, in addition to such an amount of endurance strength, an oldtime strongman, if he is a true showman, might also have some other surprising feat up his sleeve. A feat that one would not expect of a strong man to master, let alone any other person from the street, like turning a somersault in the air, doing some magic trick, speaking any provided sentence backwards, juggling, or the like.

6. An oldtime strongman is an ascetic. Being a minimalist and traditionalist, as explicated above, an oldtime strongman is tough and undemanding, like an old brewery horse. He needs generous meals to build and maintain his great strength, and to fuel his intense workouts, but, as Arthur Saxon would agree, he is able to skip a meal or two without venting the anger caused by his cramping stomach on his fellow human beings. An oldtime strongman can train and perform with the same energy in the gleaming sun or in the freezing cold. An oldtime strongman is happy with a coarse farmer's meal, and can, if necessary, sleep overnight on an old dog's blanket in the corner of a shed. An oldtime strongman takes bruises and injuries he obtained during training or performance like a man, and takes care of them quickly and properly, without any attention-getting lamentation, or a proud public display of his scars to the effects of false heroism and the inspiration of compassion. A performing oldtime strongman will not behave like a diva to his clients, he will not insist on luxuries like an opulent dressing room, fine meals, servants, or assistants. An oldtime strongman is not only actively strong, but also passively, and will bear any difficult situation stoically.

In a way, these aspects make all "contemporary" oldtime strongmen by my definition anachronistic dreamers and Romantics, naive Don Quixotes, who wish to revive long past, but in their view better and simpler, times – that is, times that, perhaps, never existed. But let us not hold them back, as we need such dreamers and idealists with a vision, who continuously and unwaveringly strive to make this world a better place, against all obvious odds and against their own deficiencies. I hope that with this book I will be able to make a small contribution to this, by offering my advice to such individuals, and by perhaps increasing their number.

3. The prerequisites to becoming an oldtime strongman and building oldtime strength

If you want to build strength like the oldtime strongmen, if you want to achieve an above-average level in some of the traditional strongman feats, or if you want to build strength on a level that makes you confident to step on a stage and do a strength performance, there are certain conditions that, if fulfilled, will help you reach such a level in the first place, or reach it faster. While there are lots of factors that will have an influence on your performance potential, most of them commonly known, there are a few that I find crucial and that are often underestimated. These are: the age at which you start lifting weights, genetic prerequisites, and willpower.

I have observed that people who start lifting weights, playing sports that demand speed and power, or doing physical work, starting from an early age, have the highest potential of building the kind of strength required for oldtime strongman work. That is, the kind of strength that lasts up to a very high age, the kind of strength that requires strong tendons and ligaments, and the kind of conditioning that makes it the most natural thing in the world for your body to perform hard physical labour. The earlier you start with regular resistance work or training, the stronger you will potentially become, and the longer you will be able to maintain your strength.

This is an observation I have made, and although I am fully convinced of it, it is rather useless and even dangerous to talk about it. This is so for several reasons. First of all, there is a huge and obvious downside to lifting weights or doing hard physical labour at a very young age, which is the risk of inhibiting bone growth or developing lasting posture problems, for example from improper lifting technique. Both of these have the unpleasant characteristic of surfacing only much later on, long after the damage has already been done.

Secondly, even if correctly done, with the proper technique, constant hard physical labour with lots of heavy lifting is still wear and tear for the body that has the potential of eventually causing problems and pain. We should not disregard the great benefits of physical activity to the human body, and its necessity for a healthy and pain-free condition, but anything that goes to extremes will take its toll sooner or later. Oldtime strongman work is, by definition, extreme, so starting with anything pertaining to that at a too early age bears the risks just described.

Thirdly, me telling you as my reader to start at the earliest possible moment, will hardly make any difference. I suppose you have already made the decision to get into oldtime strongman training quite soon and are not looking for an answer to whether you should start now or in a few years' time. Also, it is impossible to turn back the time to start earlier. So let me sum this point up by advising you to start with your oldtime strongman training right now (let us say if you are not considerably younger than eighteen years of age). If you already have long years of experience in lifting weights, in playing speed- or strength-intense sports (like track and field athletics, wrestling, climbing, etc.), or in physical labour, having started at an early age, you might have an advantage in building oldtime strength in the long run.

As a side note, weightlifting, demanding sports, and physical labour at a very early age, can also simply pertain to a childhood that is intense with age-appropriate play. Children who spend lots of time outdoors, with other children, in daylight and fresh air, in forests and fields, by riversides and on rocks, who follow their natural urge to play – playing ball, hide-and-seek, climbing trees, swimming in the lake, wrestling with each other now and then, doing acrobatics and little feats of dexterity, and engaging in creative competitions – such children will build a fantastic, natural basis for strong muscles, tendons, and ligaments in adulthood, and a robust health, in contrast to children who are forced to play indoors most of the time, in an environment that is characterised by fragile and potentially dangerous objects, limiting freedom of movement, with artificial light and artificial playmates, for example expensive toys that inhibit their creativity by dictating rules, regulations, and stories, meant to keep them busy with as little movement as possible, and to not put valuable furniture at unnecessary risk.

But let us now turn to the second aspect, the role of genetic potential in strength sports. Much has been said and written about this, especially by authors with a much more scientific approach than myself. Therefore, I do not want to add much more to the issue than two simple observations. The first observation is that I believe that yes, genetics do play a huge role in building great maximum strength. I say this because I have heard claims to the contrary, that "anyone" can become a strength athlete and reach top-level strength if they follow the right workout plan etc. While I do want to encourage anyone to work hard to reach their maximum strength potential, and while I do believe that some have managed to build incredible, live-performance-proof strength against all odds and despite mediocre genetic potential, I would never claim that some people do not have a genetic advantage over others who want to become strongmen. This would simply not be true.

If you have, by nature, strong bones, thick joints, a huge frame, and great body size or ideal leverage, and if these aspects are found throughout your family line, you will by all means have a greater potential to become a formidable strongman than someone with a naturally small frame, tender joints, and soft skin. However, it is equally true that your genetic potential cannot be modified, so spending too much words on genetic potential is equally useless as speaking too much about your potential of travelling back in time. Especially so since someone who overcomes genetic limitations is all the more admirable, and, again, I do not want, by any means, to keep you from making great strength gains despite not so ideal genetic prerequisites.

So let us instead turn towards the third aspect I mentioned, which is much less absolute, graspable, and constant: willpower. I have come to the conclusion that those who work to become strong men and women, and have more success in doing so than their fellow trainees, are those who have some kind of inner desire or motivation to work harder than anyone around them, and to stick to a regular routine without longer interruptions. This motivation and willpower can come from many different sources. Sometimes it is just inbuilt.

However, in the majority of cases, it comes from some kind of experience, like a trigger event or a persisting condition that often lies deeply buried in their subconscious. Unfortunately, I have to say that this is often a negative or sad experience. It can be anything, like having been beaten by someone larger or stronger, once or repeatedly, a generally deprived childhood, having been attacked or threatened by someone more powerful, having been left or rejected by a beloved person, having been excluded from a group, having been hugely disappointed, having had to deal with great competition, having had the feeling of one's life being on the line, or the like. Any experience like that can (but by no means has to) be the spark in a person to develop the kind of willpower and persistence to start a rigorous and highly intense training regimen and keep it up for a long enough period of time, or, in the best case, forever.

The attribute of great physical strength is something very primal and atavistic, a very basic feature that provokes highly instinctive reactive behaviour. Having lived through an experience of being threatened, belittled, or confronted with competition, can unconsciously trigger the desire and willpower to build great physical strength as a compensation. Strength gives one a natural, instinctive feeling of security, superiority, and the potential to defend oneself against future attacks. This psychological aspect of strength training is not a very pleasant topic to talk about, but let us conclude it by saying that it has at least the pleasant side of turning something bad into something good, of transforming bad energy into positive energy. This is the case if someone who has had such a negative experience starts a strength training regimen and uses his strength for the good, for example by aspiring to become a virtuous strongman according to my definition above.

To sum up, there are three not very obvious aspects that help one in becoming an unusually strong man or woman. These are: starting with resistance work at an early age, having the proper genetic potential, and having the right willpower. As the first and second aspects are in most cases given and cannot be altered (only, in the best case, overcome), you should focus on the third aspect, the willpower. Start by asking yourself if you have the motivation and unbending will to face the hard and long work it takes to conquer and perform any feat of strength that is worthy of being called such. If you have not, you can of course still follow this program to build natural and healthy physical strength, but mind you that it takes great will and endurance to do anything that goes beyond the ordinary by definition. This motivation ultimately has to come from within you and be permanent. It does not suffice if it is temporarily evoked, by looking at motivating pictures and film clips, listening to catchy slogans, or even reading a book. Not even I can provide you with this willpower. As the saying goes: I can only show you the door – you are the one who has to walk through it.

4. How I became a performing oldtime strongman

I am a performing oldtime strongman. Not only by the definition above (which, mind you, is an ideal and only formulated by myself), but also in the sense that a substantial part of my income comes from performing old-fashioned feats of strength in front of audiences on a regular basis. Thus, I am also a *professional* performing oldtime strongman – a circus artist, an entertainer, or however you want to call it. One of the questions people ask me frequently about my oldtime strongman profession is how I ended up doing this rather uncommon job in the first place. There is a short and a long version of the story.

The short version is that I started with bodybuilding training when I was 13, at home and alone, with very basic equipment. I then switched to powerlifting training when I was about 22 and had moved to Innsbruck in Austria to pursue my studies. I had by then started to regularly work out in the weight room of the sports facilities of the University of Innsbruck, and had often noticed a rather eccentric-looking man (he was only one of many eccentric people there). Wiry and athletic, with long black hair and a rugged, suntanned face, he regularly entered the weight room to do warm-up exercises that were strange and new to me.

One day he approached me and asked what sport I was training for. When I told him that I was basically only a bodybuilder, he seemed disappointed and was about to turn away. When I inquired why he had asked me this question, it turned out that he was Walter Moshammer, a former physicist from Styria, with a PhD from the University of Graz, who had worked at the CERN in Geneva and Stanford University, but had one day decided to give it all up and become an acrobat instead. He was now working full-time as a tightrope walker and handstand artist and was looking for a base to train hand to hand acrobatics. I expressed my interest and assured him that I was not only strong-looking (as he had probably expected from a bodybuilder), but also strong in actual fact. So we gave it a try and started training acrobatics. We eventually toured Germany, Austria, and Switzerland with a very simplistic acrobatic performance, for which we teamed up in between the solo performances of Walter, who would do handstands on a wobbly construction at a height of five meters, and walk tightropes ten meters above the ground without a safety net or any other precaution.

After two years of occasional shows like these, which meant a nice pocket money for a student like me, Walter, who was always a straightforward and no-nonsense person, told me that we could not go on like this. It would not pay and was becoming too strenuous for him (he was in his late forties by then), to do five or six shows a day, while I only helped in one or two of these, together with him. I would need to develop my own solo show or we could not continue working together. As I had gotten used to the extra money from these shows, I did not want to stop here.

This was the moment my stage strongman alter ego *Eisenhans* was born, and if it had not been for Walter, this would never have happened. I would also not be doing this any more, as it was also thanks to Walter's connections and network that I was able to do more and more performances per year once I had developed a solid show.

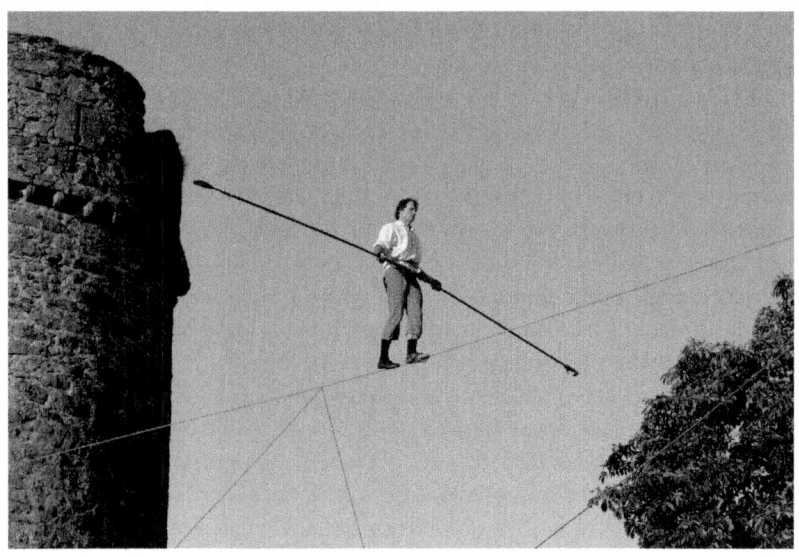

Figure 4.1 Acrobat and highwire artist Walter Moshammer from Austria.

The longer version of the story starts in my early childhood, when I impersonated the famous strongman Arthur Robin (who was recently the star of the independent Austrian-Italian film production *Mister Universo* (2016)) at the early age of three. However, I do not want to bore you with this long story, so I will close this section by summing up the most important facts: Being born to very strong parents, on the one side a sinewy mother, who, from carrying all her children and groceries for endless kilometres, had built arms that inspired the envy of her own son, and on the other side a broad-shouldered father with a tremendous amount of natural strength, honed in post-war Germany by training with bricks, for the lack of any other possibility, and after a very active and adventurous childhood full of play outdoors, and deprived of the straight jacket of any regulated training in any popular sport, I started out as a bodybuilder by my own decision at a very young age, then turned to powerlifting, and then, by chance, after a short detour into hand to hand acrobatics, I ended up, quite suddenly and out of necessity, as a performing oldtime strongman.

I then took some time to prepare my first few shows. They consisted of the following feats: driving a spike through a wooden board, bending a nail, tearing a deck of cards, teeth lifting a large wooden barrel filled with various weights, and the bed-of-nails and anvil trick, where you lie down on a bed of nails, let an anvil be placed on your chest, and ask someone from the audience to hit the anvil with a large sledgehammer (The latter, by the way, is not really a feat of strength. It can be performed by anyone with some courage and pain tolerance, but it makes for a good effect – although it is also quite dangerous).

Over the years I then continuously worked on my show and reputation in three ways: 1) I improved my strength performance, working my way up the ladder towards tougher nails, horseshoes, decks of cards, etc. step by step. 2) I worked on my show, the way it is structured, the way I present the feats, etc. 3) I worked on achieving certain bench marks of strength that would provide proof for my real-world strength (I still continue to do so). Here are some of my achievements:

- Lifting the Dinnie Stones without lifting straps or belt
- Lifting and shouldering the Inver Stone and holding it with one hand
- Officially bending the Ironmind Red Nail
- Bending a Kerckhaert sx7 horseshoe, size 000, beyond 180 degrees
- Closing the Ironmind #3 hand gripper with a 30mm (1.1in) set
- Lifting 90kg (200lbs) on a Rolling Thunder deadlift handle
- Teeth lifting 100kg (221lbs)
- Squatting 230kg (500lbs) raw in competition
- Bench pressing 180kg (397lbs) raw in competition
- Deadlifting 287.5kg (635lbs) raw in competition
- Deadlifting 220kg (486lbs) with a four-finger grip (index and middle fingers, reverse grip)
- Deadlifting 140kg (309lbs) with a two-finger grip (middle fingers only, reverse grip)

5. Run, throw, lift, climb: How I divide the body into movement functions

So how did I (and still do) go about building and maintaining strength for my shows, and how should one train his body to develop oldtime strength? For a start, I would like to go back in time even a bit further than the period from the late 1800s to the early twentieth century, the period that I call the golden age of the strongmen. I would like to go back to a period that was, in many ways, a romanticized ideal to which these old-time strongmen aspired: antiquity.

Our modern idea of sports in the Western world originated in Greek antiquity, and in the original Olympic games. The earliest disciplines of the Olympic games were running, then jumping, throwing the javelin, throwing the discus, and wrestling, later also boxing, and even later chariot races and pankration (a combination of different martial arts techniques). This appears like an arbitrary choice of sports, a choice of sports the Greeks were incidentally aware of. But if we look at it more closely, we realize two things: These disciplines were 1) very basic movements, at first sight war-like, but at second sight simply 2) necessary for human survival since prehistoric times.

To realize this, we might want to go back in time even farther, and look at prehistory in more detail. Two particular anthropological features of anatomically modern humans and related human species, like the Neanderthals, are the upright walk (as opposed to quadrupedalism) and the use of tools. Also, it is accepted as a fact nowadays that the gradual increase in size and capability of the pre-human brain was connected to an increase of protein-rich foods, i.e. mostly animal foods – probably starting with fish and eventually pertaining to big game that had to be hunted down in a complexly arranged and well-cooperating social group, and with the help of tools.

Now, looking again at the earliest organized sporting event in history, the original Olympic games, we realize the atavistic quality and symbolism of the Greek disciplines: running and jumping – the amplified test of the most basic human movement (the upright walk) and the prerequisite to any successful hunt; throwing the javelin and discus – the most basic use of tools to hunt down big game, i.e. throwing a potentially lethal weapon; wrestling – a competition that not only tests and builds overall strength and martial skill effectively, but that is also designed for a determination of ranks within a complex social group, like a group of hunters, without losing any good hunter through lethal injury. (This is, by the way, the major difference between wrestling and boxing: if one simply wants a fair competition to determine who is stronger, they wrestle. If one wants to destroy his opponent, they box. It must be owed to the increasingly war-like culture of the ancient Greeks that boxing was eventually added to the Olympic disciplines.) These basic disciplines – *running, jumping, throwing,* and *wrestling* – are so primeval and basically human that you encounter them in almost any aboriginal culture in some form of sporting event.

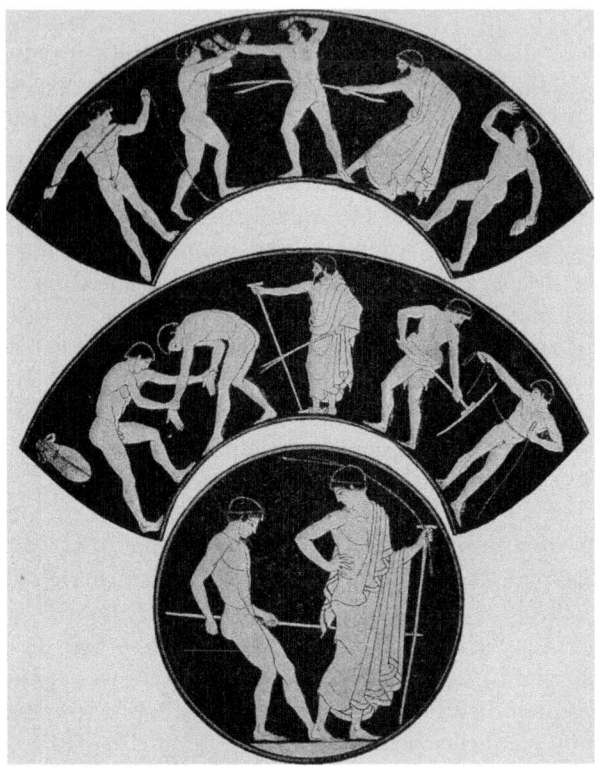

Figure 5.1 Sportsmen in ancient Greece.

Next, there are further basic human movements for which we can trace the origin in (cultural) anthropology. I already talked about the upright walk as a typical human trait. According to one theory, it bears witness to the gradual adaptation to a life on the ground, in the African Savannah, in contrast to a life in the trees. As a result of this change, humans became inferior climbers compared to our primate relatives, and nobody would deny that any chimpanzee could beat us humans at a tree-climbing match. Even if some of us manage to build amazing climbing skills in the courses of our lives, and great strength in our hands and back muscles, it is a commonly known fact that apes have much stronger hand and arm muscles by nature. However, the observation that we humans have *lost* so much in terms of climbing skills suggests by implication that we *stem from* a tree-climbing species, and obviously we have not lost *all* of our climbing skills. Also, climbing was, throughout human history, always a means to *gather* additional food sources that complement hunting – fruit, nuts, honey, etc. In short, *climbing* is still a basic human skill.

Next, there are two further, related movements that humans are particular suited to perform, which are *lifting and carrying*. By lifting, in this context, I mean particularly lifting to hip-height, like in a deadlift, or at most chest- or shoulder-height, but not so much overhead lifting. Both lifting and carrying are closely connected to the primeval developments I already talked about. Let us again imagine the scenario of a prehistoric big game hunt: humans are organized in a coordinated group of hunters that runs after a large mammal and tracks it down (upright walk, running, jumping). The hunters pick up stones and use primitive spears and throw them after the animal to hurt and weaken it (throwing). The animal collapses, comes to lie on the ground, and a few of the strongest hunters lift huge boulders to eventually kill it (lifting). The animal is butchered with simple stone tools, and the hunters lift up the parts to carry them to their base, perhaps a large cave, where the rest of the tribe welcomes the hunters and their prey (lifting and carrying).

On a less speculative level, many human cultures around the world in fact had or still have a tradition of lifting stones to test and train their strength, and to establish a social hierarchy. Scottish and Icelandic lifting stones, like the Inver Stone or the Husafell Stone, are relatively recent and popular examples, but also the Basque lifting stones provide proof for this basic human tradition. In Japan, a friend of mine discovered two lifting stones with a display board that said:

> "*Ban-mochi Ishi*: This stone was once used to see who is the strongest in a village.
> Sometimes people lifted up rice bags for the measurement, and sometimes they used heavy rocks like these. Its round shape was suitable since not only arm strength but also grip strength is required to lift it up. The bigger stone weighs 25Kan (93.75kg [207lbs]), the smaller one weighs 20Kan (75kg [166lbs])."

But also the ancient Greeks apparently lifted stones to impress and set superlatives. Several stones have been found with inscriptions dating to Greek antiquity, documenting the styles in which they were lifted and the names of the lifters. Although these stones, weighing from 45kg (99lbs) to 480kg (1,060lbs), leave some doubt as to the lifting technique, as to whether the inscriptions document actual feats of strength or fantasy, and as to whether the inscriptions really refer to the inscribed stones themselves and not to other stones, they doubtlessly prove that the ancient Greeks were interested in stone lifting as a test of strength.

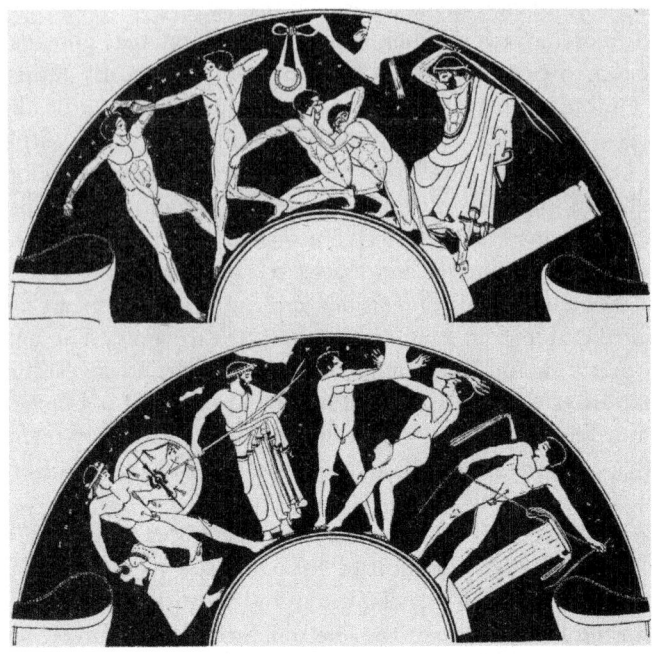

Figure 5.2 Greek martial artists in antiquity.

Although stone lifting (or simply heavy-object-lifting, for that matter) and stone carrying was never as well established and institutionalized as other basic sports (that is, until the invention of weightlifting as a competitive sport in the course of the golden age of the strongmen), it served many ancient cultures as a similar competition to establish ranks as wrestling: a friendly contest that tests and trains muscular strength in the members of a group or tribe, without burning them out, or risking fatal injury. In sum, I argue that *lifting and carrying* are very basic human movements as well.

Then there is another form of human movement that evolved with the use of tools, which is *hitting*. By hitting I mean *hitting with a tool*, not hitting with the arms, hands or fists, which I count to *boxing*. While we might argue that throwing a stone is the most basic, particularly human use of a tool, a close consideration suggests that hitting is not a long way away from it, and might have evolved simultaneously, or, perhaps, even earlier. We know that there are many primates who use stones or pieces of wood as a sort of hammer to open nuts or fruit, and it can most easily be imagined that early humans did the same.

Further down the line, the earliest preserved human tools, hand axes, are proof of the use of tools for *hitting* (although they were in time probably also used for *cutting* motions). But also pieces of wood, if not used as spears, can be used as clubs to kill or weaken an animal. Once you have invented and built a primitive stone axe with a wooden handle, you can use it to cut down trees in a hitting motion.

Of course, all of these tools, and also simple wooden sticks, can also be used to hurt fellow human beings, for example in a stick-fighting contest – the earliest form of fencing. The practice of some primates to pull large branches of trees through the jungle, and wave them about which large noise and havoc to impress their fellow tribal members, is not a long way from this.

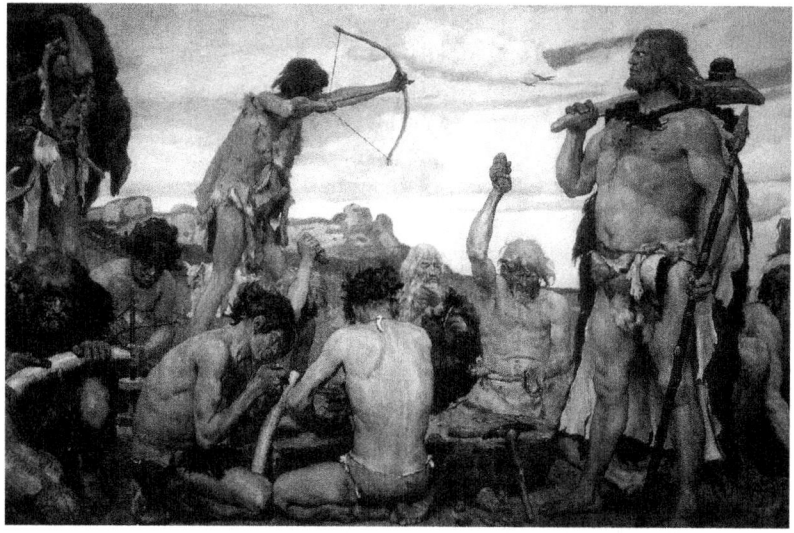

Figure 5.3 Palaeolithic activities ("Stone Age" by Viktor Vasnetsov).

To sum up, I believe that there is only a limited number of original human "sports", and all of them relate to, or replicate, basic human movements that were necessary for the survival of early mankind, as it had evolved from its ancestors. These are *running and jumping, throwing, wrestling, climbing,* and *lifting and carrying*. In the long run, a few other sports eventually added to this, with the advent of certain basic human inventions and cultural achievements – and the increasing drive to wage wars, probably connected to the rise of agriculture, which again lead to the concept of private property (especially in the form of land and livestock) and an increase in population. These include (not in any speculative chronological order): *boxing, hitting* (including fencing or stick fighting), *shooting* (first with the bow and arrow), *horse riding* (with the taming of horses in the aftermath of the agricultural revolution), *swimming* (once humans had overcome their fear of water), any form of *paddling and rowing* in a primitive boat once such had been invented (e.g. the dugout, the kayak, and the canoe), and, one might argue, *dancing* (to add something a bit more cheerful).

If you now take any kind of physical sport humans like to play today, you will be able to trace it back to these basic human movements. *Hiking* is nothing but walking, and thus a sort of a basis, and not even a sport in the closest sense. As my remarks above have shown, the *track and field* disciplines, including the *sprint*, the *decathlon*, the *steeplechase*, the *throwing events*, etc., are the most basic and original form of sports. Any form of regulated *wrestling* follows soon after that, whether it be Sumo wrestling, Turkish oil wrestling, the Alpine *Ranggeln*, the Swiss *Schwingen*, Graeco-Roman wrestling, or any other of the scores of different existing forms of this sport. *Soccer*, for example, involves mostly running, but also illustrates an interesting aspect that many team sports feature, which is the simple imitation of a hunt, with the necessity of strategic cooperation within a familiar group, and with a prey. In this case it is a little round leather ball, which seems to replicate a small defenceless animal, like a fox, rabbit, or perhaps a flightless bird.

Also, team events nicely illustrate the aspect of the imitation of war that many sports have incorporated in the course of time, as one group of players fights another, often despised, group. *Rugby, American football*, and *basketball* are obviously comparable to soccer here, although they are a bit more complex, as they also incorporate the movement pattern of *throwing*. *Cricket* and *baseball* include a form of *hitting* with a tool, a bat, instead. The same is true for *tennis, badminton,* and related sports, minus the group aspect.

Any kind of *race*, be it with a motorcar, motorcycle, or bicycle, is simply a further development of the *horse race,* whether with a rider or a cart, which in itself is only an amplified version of a run. *Weightlifting, powerlifting* and the modern *strongman* sport (to return to the closer context of the premise of this book) are obviously more or less complex forms of *lifting* (and *carrying*). Although *bodybuilding* training is similar to weightlifting training, the sport itself, if a sport at all, is hard to pin down. One must come to the conclusion that it probably derives from some form of *dance*, like other disciplines that are judged by aesthetic criteria, like *figure skating*, and, of course, *ballroom dancing*. Hunting is obviously a very original sport, although nowadays it almost exclusively incorporates *shooting*, rather than *throwing*.

Other animal sports in which the animal is not killed immediately, but only once it is burned out, are mostly forms of *horse riding* or *chariot racing*, or primeval form of this, reminiscent of the process of overcoming the fear of, domesticating, and taming large mammals like horses. These include the *rodeo* and *sled dog racing* (arguably even older than the horse race). *Boxing* is boxing, and *fencing* is fencing, that is, *hitting*. *Climbing* as a basic human movement is arguably under-represented in popular sports today, perhaps for the reasons explicated above: that is was originally a human feature to emancipate ourselves from the dependency of trees and the climbing of them. However, ever since the birth of *mountaineering*, climbing has experienced a renaissance in the form of *rock climbing*. Mountaineering leads me to *skiing*, which is *ski touring* (which is walking with a form of snow shoes) minus the touring. *Cross-country skiing* is running or walking, depending on the intensity.

Talking about cross-country skiing: where it gets interesting are those disciplines that are some form of combination of several disciplines, like the *biathlon,* which combines *cross-country skiing* (running) with shooting. Such sports nicely illustrate the original, life-relevant quality of institutionalized sports, that is, their origin in the hunt for food, and/or war. *Modern pentathlon*, a relatively little-known sport, is an even nicer illustration and very basic and universal, as it also combines running with shooting, and adds to that horse riding, fencing, and swimming. The *Scottish Highland Games* traditionally consist of all sorts of throwing events (logs, stones...), but also track and field disciplines like a steeplechase and the running of different distances. However, one need not necessarily look at institutionalized sports to find such disciplines combined. In medieval Europe, the concept of institutionalized sports as in ancient Greece did no longer exist in the minds of the population, but nevertheless, aspiring knights regularly trained their horse riding, fencing, throwing, and bow-and-arrow skills, and organized tournaments to test and train their martial skill. In his juvenile adventure stories of Robin Hood, Howard Pyle paints a romantic picture of the Merry Men spending their time in the Sherwood forest with "bouts of wrestling", "cudgel play", "bouts at quarterstaff", and "shooting at garlands hung upon a willow wand."

In sum, any kind of sport originates in one form or the other from very few basic human movement patterns. There are only very few exceptions, for example chess, which is more of a mental than a physical challenge, or curling (I do not mean the curling of a dumbbell or barbell, but the discipline in the Olympic Winter Games), which is a movement remotely reminiscent of *throwing*, but combined with other movements apparently derived from doing household chores. Here, I would like to list the basic human movement patterns again, according to two categories.

First, the more basic ones:

1. Walking, running, and jumping
2. Throwing
3. Climbing
4. Lifting and carrying
5. Hitting
6. Wrestling

And second, the more specialized movements, which required further cultural achievements:

1. Boxing
2. Shooting
3. Horse riding
4. Swimming
5. Paddling
6. Dancing

Of course, the human body is very versatile and able to do a lot more different movements, like, for example, *crawling*, or *pulling* and *pushing* movements, etc. However, I believe my list is complete in terms of basic movements where humans were always pushed to maximum performance to ensure survival in a complex group (hunting, gathering and preparing food, establishing a hierarchy, self-defence, etc.).

Let us now return to oldtime strongman training and how all of the issues above fit into this topic. It seems that weightlifting, powerlifting, the modern strongman sport, and thus probably also oldtime strongman training, are simply disciplines that correspond most closely to the basic human movement pattern of *lifting*. However, earlier on, in one of my introductory chapters, I argued that a true oldtime strongman is a universalist, an athlete who strives towards a wide array of skills and overall strength in a large variety of movements. Thus, I approach the property of being an oldtime strongman, and my oldtime strongman training, with more than just one basic human movement pattern in mind. Ideally, an oldtime strongman incorporates *all* of the basic human movement patterns into his training, or at least perceives his training as *derived* from all of them. What I mean is that a *complete* training and development of the human body, if there is such a thing, must result from replicating at least the *entire* first, the *basic* category of human movement patterns.

The more specialized second category might be excluded, although it would of course be nice if someone were well versed in these skills as well. Would you not agree that an athlete who is a great runner, jumper, thrower, climber, lifter, hitter, and wrestler, is a very complete athlete? And an even better one if he could also box, ride, shoot, swim, paddle, and dance? I think yes. This is so for the obvious reason that if one trained all of these disciplines, he would automatically train all the muscles in his body: running and jumping trains the legs, throwing trains the shoulders and chest, climbing trains the upper back, biceps and grip, lifting trains the lower back and grip as well, hitting trains the core, and wrestling trains all of these muscle groups in combination.

This is what I believe you should ideally strive for when you decide to start with oldtime strongman training. There were, in fact, oldtime strongmen of the golden age who perfectly personified this ideal. The most splendid example is the Scotsman Donald Dinnie, who was an unbeaten Highland Games champion, which means he was a great thrower, but he was also a track and field champion, a successful wrestler, and he lifted and carried the Dinnie Stones, thus writing oldtime strongman and stonelifting history.

Of course, not everyone has the time and means to train all of the above disciplines simultaneously. But what most people will want to do at least is to replicate the basic human movement patterns with dumbbell- and barbell training, and a basic weightlifting routine that trains the whole body. Now you might say that this is what most strength athletes do any way, so what were all these complicated expositions for?

First of all, I wanted you to realize where all the exercises originated that we perform to train our bodies, and what the original purposes of our locomotor system were. Secondly, I believe it is a difference whether you image, or visualize, simply that you, for example, *train your shoulders* when you lift a barbell overhead, or whether this motion actually replicates *throwing*. In this sense, every exercise you perform should be chosen and performed with the basic human movement pattern that it replicates in mind. This will automatically lead you towards becoming a great all-round athlete and strongman.

Instead of simply *doing pull-ups*, you remind yourself that this is a replication of *climbing*. Instead of simply *doing a deadlift*, you train to *lift* a huge stone. Instead of simply *doing squats*, you train the muscles needed for high *jumps* and fast *runs*. I am not saying that you ultimately will have to climb a tree or go out and sprint (although it cannot hurt), but I am saying that you should constantly remind yourself of what you body was designed for, and where we humans come from.

I have, however, two more aspects for you to consider, as there are two more movements, or movement patterns, humans were designed for. These are *biting* and *dexterity*. Let me talk about biting first. Yes, you read correctly. I would like to consider biting a specific human skill, although it is by no means a particularly well-developed skill in anatomically modern humans. On the contrary, rather like climbing, it is one of the skills we humans unlearned bit by bit and keep doing so drastically, in particular since the advent of agriculture. In relation to our body weight, our biting skills are quite underdeveloped in comparison to most mammals in the animal kingdom. Nevertheless, we have not yet lost them completely. Our muscles of mastication include some of the strongest muscles in the human body in relation to their size, and considering the small leverage of your jawbone, it is incredible what these muscles can do when one comes to think of it. The mouth, with jaw and teeth, was an irreplaceable tool (and weapon, for that matter) for early humans, who, for example, tightened animal skins by holding them with their teeth to tan them, or chewed the skins for the same purpose. Also, a mere look into the animal kingdom will demonstrate that it is the most natural thing in the world to put jaw and neck muscles under severe stress – just imagine a cheetah dragging its prey up into a tree top, or the legendary bite force of hyenas.

It is a commonly known fact that humans in primal cultures had much better developed jawbones – large enough to fit all teeth comfortably in – and teeth, before they underwent a civilization process after contact with the Western world. Nowadays, dentists generously deal out braces, and seem to have a strong motivation to ensure that every human being has at least once in their life been tortured by such a device. In so-called civilized cultures it is an everyday phenomenon, yes, even an expectation for children to have all sorts of problems with malpositioned teeth, because the teeth do not fit into their underdeveloped jawbones. These problems seem to be nutrition-related, apparently also connected to a lack of certain micronutrients, but, more obviously, also to the softness of our foods. In particular products from processed grain, but any processed foods in general, are exceedingly soft. I strongly believe that our jaws and teeth lack the sort of challenge the chewing of *natural* foods generates. They are challenged too little. Muscles, bones, and tendons (it is tendons that hold our teeth in place) need stress to grow thick and strong. Practically no modern human maxes out the great working potential of our jaw muscles.

You probably already sense what my point is. It was a particular asset of the oldtime strongmen to display feats of teeth strength (not all – Hermann Görner considered them silly) and I am no exception. But, as opposed to what most people say or think when they see a feat of teeth strength – that it is risky and dangerous, even foolish, or at best odd, to try to lift a weight by the teeth – I think it would be beneficial to most people's health to challenge their jaw muscles from time to time, at least more so than people from the street commonly do. Please do not get me wrong. The sort of extreme feats some oldtime strongmen performed and perform are indeed risky. One must be extremely cautious when trying to replicate something of this kind. All I am saying is that in principle, our jaws and teeth can handle a much greater load than what most people would image. I will talk more about feats of teeth strength later. For now, let me summarize that biting is a skill that is essentially and naturally human as well, and can be trained like any of the skills mentioned above if one desires to do so.

The next skill, or set of movement patterns, is even more particularly human. This is *dexterity*. As humans are the most efficient and creative tool users on the planet, they have, through the process of evolution, developed hands that are extremely versatile and have almost unlimited possibilities of manipulating objects. They can grab all sorts of objects, they can crush objects, hold onto objects, twist objects, and so on. Using one's hands in a great variety of ways is indisputably human and should be trained by any oldtime strongman with a wide range of grip and wrist strength exercises.

With these amendments, let me once more sum up what an oldtime strongman should strive for. To become a complete athlete, one should make sure to replicate all of the following basic (groups of) human movement patterns in his training:

1. Walking, running, and jumping
2. Throwing
3. Climbing
4. Lifting and carrying
5. Hitting
6. Biting
7. Dexterity

As you can see, I have excluded wrestling, because, although wrestling is a fantastic full body workout, the other movements cover all of the muscles in the body already. Also, it is not possible for everyone to incorporate wrestling sessions into his busy schedule in addition to his weightlifting training, and wrestling bears a high risk for injuries. However, many of the oldtime strongmen of the golden age have engaged in wrestling (and many of the great wrestlers of that time were also strongmen – the transitions between a good wrestler and a good strongman were fluent). One reason for this was that many strongmen would typically be challenged to enter into wrestling matches, or would even offer this opportunity to their audiences themselves to demonstrate their strength. Last but not least, wrestling skills can be used for self-defence purposes, and it does not have to be Graeco-Roman wrestling, but can be any other form of this sport.

To conclude these expositions on human movement patterns, I want you to keep in mind where we humans come from, how the architecture of our bodies evolved, and what our human locomotor system is designed for. If we remember this, we will be able to devise a workout plan accordingly, to become as versatile and complete an athlete as possible, and, although the effect will probably not be so different to that of any workout plan that trains all the muscles in the body, it will keep us rooted in our human physiology.

6. Developing overall strength: Finding exercises to build your whole body

Now, based on these findings, there are obviously several methods to train your body to cover all of the basic movements and movement patterns. The most obvious approach will be with barbells and dumbbells – the classic tools of the oldtime strongman – and I will give you a simple example for this.

1. Walking, running, and jumping: To train these movements, an oldtime strongman should first of all make sure to walk a lot. This will appear counter-intuitive to you, but I firmly believe that walking is the basis of any athletic body and a necessary means to keep healthy and fit. Regular hikes and long walks, or at least a regular walk to the bus station twice a day, and some stairs taken during the day, should be part of any strongman's daily routine, or, for that matter, of any human. Beyond this, you should obviously perform some heavy barbell lifting with exercises like back squats, front squats, lunges, etc. to replicate the basic running and jumping movements. However, for an oldtime strongman workout you might also want to look into exercises that enable you to move a little more weight, like the back lift, feet balancing feats, squats with a limited range of motion, or supporting feats.

2. Throwing: When you throw an object, you push it away from the body. Thus, barbell exercises that replicate throwing will be such that imitate a pushing motion, like the military shoulder press, the push press, overhead triceps extensions, or the bench press. Overhead pressing should be part of an oldtime strongman's routine any way, in particular the military shoulder press, the push press, and the one-hand push press, as these are some of the most classic feats of strength. However, this has somewhat become the speciality of the Olympic weightlifters, who clean and jerk such incredible weights that hardly anyone will be impressed by what a universalist, who trains many different disciplines at the same time, will be able to achieve. The same is true for the log press of the modern strongmen, which is a nice variation – one I would encourage any aspiring oldtime strongman to try some day. Ideally, though, you will find some more unusual exercise to shine, like, for example, kettlebell juggling (which is very old-school and very closely connected to the human movement of throwing), limited range of motion overhead lifts, or some of the wonderful Scottish Highland Games disciplines, which are literally and in the most traditional sense, "throws". Talking about kettlebells: kettlebell swings themselves are a wonderful exercise to train the muscles in you body needed for throwing objects upwards (although some people have

tried to sell this exercise as some mysterious, almost magic, full-body workout, whereas it is not much more than a throwing motion that naturally involves several muscles in the body, as most of the original human movement patterns do).

3. Climbing: Although actual, real-life climbing of a tree, rock, etc. involves many different muscles groups, including the legs and chest, most people will agree that climbing requires strong back, biceps, and hand muscles first and foremost. Therefore, climbing can most easily be replicated by pull-ups. This is an exercise everyone should include in his regimen by any means – if not for performance reasons, then at least to make sure the spine is stretched regularly, in particular in consideration of all the heavy lifting an oldtime strongman has to do. If you are lightweight, you can amplify your pull-ups by attaching additional weight to your belt to increase the effect of stretching the spine. There is a way climbing can be replicated by this exercise for wonderful feats of strength, which are pull-ups, made more difficult by additional grip challenges. You can do pull-ups with all sorts of limitations, e.g. with only one arm, or with two arms but only one or two fingers per hand, on a very narrow edge with your fingertips only, on ropes or towels, on very thick bars, and so on. Incidentally, you do not need to buy any fancy equipment for this, as mostly all of these possibilities can be improvised with very simple means. Even if you do not train for such a feat with the aim of performing it live, you can consider such exercises part of your grip strength training.

4. Lifting and carrying: This is where an oldtime strongman will have to do lots of heavy work. The most obvious barbell exercise here is the deadlift, but I also consider barbell rowing as lifting, and under certain circumstances even biceps curls. Thus, besides the spinal erectors, I consider the latissimus and biceps muscles essential to the lifting and carrying movement patterns as well. On a more specialized oldtime strongman level, there are loads of lifting and carrying feats you can train for. A beautiful and very primal feat of strength is obviously the lifting of a heavy stone. This can also be extended to carrying the stone across a certain distance. I should probably mention the classic and world famous lifting stones like the Inver Stone, the Dinnie Stones, or the Husafell Stone here, but I want to talk about these in more detail later. Also, you have the option of training with, and lifting, the so-called Atlas Stones that modern strongmen use, made of concrete and having a spherical shape. But although these offer a quite interesting challenge, it is more pleasing to the eye to witness a man lifting an irregular, natural stone. These can offer a greater variety of challenges, from a particularly slippery, to a craggy surface, or from a particularly condense, to an irregular, unwieldy shape. But lifting feats do

not stop here. You can train towards a heavy harness or hip lift, if you find a belt or harness suitable for this. In these movements you will be able to lift astronomical weights. Or, you could train on variations of the deadlift, for example with grip variations (one hand, two fingers, four fingers...), or train for a one-finger lift, the speciality of the famous Bavarian oldtime strongman Hans Steyrer. Along these lines there are lots of grip strength feats that are lifts in the closest sense, and I will talk more about these later.

5. Hitting: You were probably already wondering how you should train for the hitting movement. In essence, one characteristic of any effective and aptly violent hitting motion is that it trains the core, the abdominal muscles (although the latissimus muscle and others are also stressed). Depending on whether the hitting motion is more of a straight, downward motion, along a vertical axis, a sideways motion on a horizontal axis, or a diagonal motion performed across the front of the body, different sections of the straight or oblique abdominal muscles, that is, of the *musculus rectus abdominis*, respectively *musculus obliquus externus abdominis*, are involved.

While most people nowadays would not consider training these muscles with an actual hitting motion, there is such a possibility indeed: hitting a large rubber loader tyre with a sledgehammer. Hitting this tire with a downward, vertical motion, or a sideways, horizontal motion, are fantastic exercises for the core. Also, you can perform similar movements on a cable tower, holding onto the cable with almost any handle and performing hitting motions, as if you were holding an axe to chop wood or to cut down a tree.

However, most will be satisfied with the results of traditional abdominal exercises. As oldtime strongmen need a particular strong core for all sorts of feats, these traditional exercises, like the prototypical sit-up, should preferably be performed with additional weight, rather than with the high numbers of repetitions some trainees commonly perform. One a side note, because of the particular necessity of a strong core for oldtime strongmen, you should be prepared to develop a strong-*looking* core as well. By this I do not mean so much the visible vertical and horizontal separations along the straight abdominal muscles, but a somewhat *thicker* core than what a mere bodybuilder, someone who trains mostly for optical reasons, would probably desire. The priority of as thin and slender a waist as possible in proportion to the shoulder-width, is something an aspiring oldtime strongman should do away with. He should trade it for the priority of a core and waist that *are* actually strong, and expect to sacrifice some of the visually pleasing V-shape for this.

Coming back to ways of training the hitting movement, there is a classic strongman feat that requires such. This is the feat of driving a nail into, or through, a wooden board without a hammer, merely by holding it in one's fist. There are some variations to this feat, for example using a very large spike instead of a rather common, smaller nail, or driving it through car license plates instead of – or in addition to – a piece of wood. Any variation is a very impressing feat of strength. It has the advantage that audiences can relate to it really well, as most people have tried to hammer a nail into a board at least once in their lives. It is also one of the few regularly performed oldtime strongman feats that actually replicate a hitting motion. Other feats exist, but they seem to belong to the realm of karate and other martial arts, like breaking boards and bricks with bare hands.

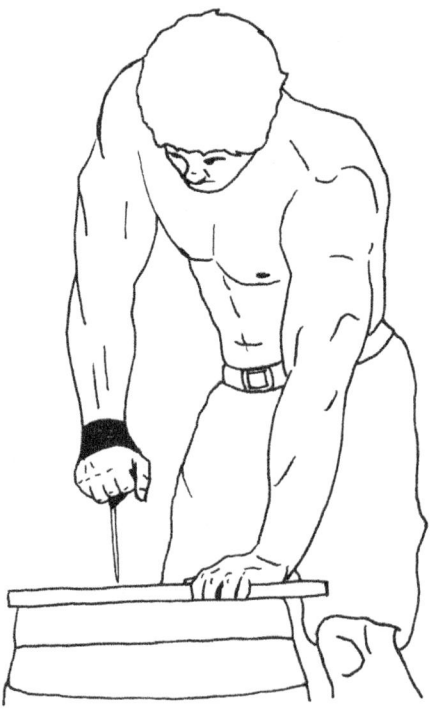

Figure 6.1 Getting ready for nail driving.

However, there are more strongman feats that, although they do not replicate a hitting motion, require some of the muscle groups of this movement pattern. These are, mostly, braced steel bending feats. Braced bending means that you bend the steel against a point of resistance on your body, most commonly your thigh, although it can also be your knee, hip, head, neck, etc. The sort of feats where you, for example, push a steel bar downward, with its centre resting against your thigh, require a strong effort from the core, and a flexing of the abdominal muscles. The same is true for horseshoe bending – one of the best, classic oldtime strongman feats. Horseshoe bending requires a lot of strength from the hands and wrists, but also a particular surge of power from the core.

6. Biting: The beauty of teeth strength feats is that they do not only train the jaw muscles, but also the neck. Thus, any training of your neck muscles can be considered part of your oldtime strongman training, whether you do it with the aim of performing teeth strength feats or not. There are also, by the way, feats of strength where you lift objects with your head, by using a special harness. This requires strong neck muscles, but not your jaw. However, although great loads of weight can potentially be lifted in this manner, pure head lifting feats are not as visually pleasing and impressing.

So, again, let us assume that you do not plan to perform teeth strength feats, but you want to be a complete athlete. Then you could train your jaw muscles simply by chewing tough meals now and then, and by not avoiding foods like raw carrots, nuts, tough or dried meat, etc. In addition to this, you could train your neck muscles like wrestlers and boxers commonly do, with wrestler's bridges in all directions. If you do these in a backward motion, with your back pointing towards the floor, you will realize how strong the human neck actually is, or how much potential it has. I regularly performed this exercise with several 20kg (44lbs) plates of additional weight on my belly, before I even started with oldtime strongman training. However, the muscles on the front of the neck are not as strong.

If you do decide to get into training for teeth strength feats, you are well advised to go about it very cautiously. The weak link in such feats is probably the teeth themselves, which are not naturally replaceable or repairable. Therefore, it goes without saying that you should always protect your teeth with some kind of padding, like a robust cloth. I strongly prefer leather, although others have used various kinds of artificial fabric very efficiently. Also, your fragile cervical spine is always in danger when doing teeth strength feats, so do not take them lightly! The other side of the coin is, however, that strong neck muscles actually *protect* you cervical spine in everyday life. This you should consider.

There are a number of common feats of teeth strength. The teeth lift is the most basic and straightforward exercise and goes a long way. You can lift a maximum weight, you can lift a weight for repetitions, you can lift people, etc. A very similar stress on your jaw, but actually a bit more comfortable, because it reduces stress on the spine, is the motion of towing something with your teeth, like a car. This is to many a very impressive feat, although towing a modern car with your teeth, on a road without a slope, is the easiest thing in the world. I have on one occasion towed three cars in a row and on another occasion a horse cart with a musical band on it, and both were no real challenge.

Next in line are steel bending feats with your teeth. The most popular version of this is bending a steel bar by holding it in your jaw (with a piece of cloth wrapped around it, of course) in the centre, and your hands at the ends of the bar. There are limitations to how much you can bend in this manner, but the fact that you hold the bar in your mouth, makes up for this with a great show effect.

Then, you can bend almost anything with your teeth if the object is fixed in a vice: from nails, across horseshoes and wrenches, to coins. Depending on your technique, you can train slightly different muscles in your neck with these, for example if you bite onto it with your front teeth or your back teeth.

Last but not least, there are balancing feats, where you hold or carry a visually appealing object in your mouth, like a chair or a table. I will talk more about teeth strength feats and the training for it below.

7. Dexterity: This is synonymous with grip and wrist strength, and any oldtime strongman should put a great focus on this in his training. The large majority of feats of strength that differentiate the classic oldtime strongmen from the modern weightlifters, powerlifters, and strongmen either have to do with grip, wrist, or teeth strength. The beauty about grip strength also seems to be that drugs, which usually help with the increase of muscle mass and overall strength, and thus offer a welcomed short-cut to some modern-day trainees, do not seem to help so much in developing greater grip strength than outstanding natural athletes can achieve. Proof for this may be sought in some of the truly great grip strength legends, who either lived before the advent of these unpleasant aids, or evade suspicion because of their relatively average appearance and body composition, like Joe Kinney. There is a vast multitude of grip and wrist strength exercises, and I not want to talk about all of them here – first, because I will talk more about them below, and second, because I have written a whole book about this, to which I would like to refer you. It is called *Grip Strength* and I have written it together with the American Tommy Heslep, also one of the truly great grip strength athletes alive (and also a natural athlete). For now, I only want to emphasize that grip and wrist strength exercises are a must for any aspiring oldtime strongman and should be a fixed component of your training regimen.

As you can see, you can make your choice of whether you want to cover a movement pattern by a simple and basic barbell exercise, or whether you want to cover it by training for some beautiful and seldom seen feat of strength as you go along. In any case, and once more, I strongly advise you to cover all of the basic movement patterns above in your workout, even if you do it with unevenly distributed intensity. One reason for this is that you should avoid an imbalance in your body, as this can lead to pain and injuries. Any of the basic movement patterns can be turned into a feat of strength, but none has to. Thus, the possibilities of combination for an oldtime strongman training regimen are endless. The way your workout plan will look also depends on your desired area of specialization and your current focus – things I will talk about in more detail below.

To conclude this section, I will give you another clear overview of some basic exercises that, in combination, will build strength in your whole body (I do not mention particular feats of strength here yet, as I will talk about these in a later section). Mind you that this is only a selection and that many of these exercises have different variations as well, which I do not list here in their entirety:

1. Walking, running, and jumping:
   ♦ Hiking, trail running, cross-country skiing, sprinting, track and field disciplines (hurdles, long jump, high jump...)
   ♦ Squats, front squats, lunges, leg presses, Hackenschmidt squats ("hack squats"), leg extensions, leg curls, calf raises

2. Throwing:
   ♦ Shot put, hammer throwing, spear throwing, discus throwing, Highland Games disciplines (putting the stone, tossing the caber, weight for height...)
   ♦ Shoulder press, push press, clean and jerk, snatch
   ♦ Bench press
   ♦ Triceps extension
   ♦ Kettlebell exercises (swings, cleans, snatch, juggling...)

3. Climbing
   ♦ Rock climbing, rope climbing
   ♦ Pull-ups
   ♦ Latissimus pull-downs on a cable tower

4. Lifting and carrying
- ◆ Stonelifting and -carrying
- ◆ Deadlifts
- ◆ Bent-over rows
- ◆ Rows on a cable tower
- ◆ Upright rows
- ◆ Biceps curls
- ◆ Farmers walk

5. Hitting
- ◆ Cricket, baseball, chopping wood, sword and stick fighting
- ◆ Sledgehammer swings
- ◆ Abdominal exercises

6. Biting
- ◆ Chewing tough foods
- ◆ Wrestler's bridges in all directions

7. Dexterity
- ◆ Basic exercises for other movement patterns with wrist and grip emphasis (reverse biceps curls, hammer curls, triceps extension behind the head with a dumbbell, climbing and lifting exercises with more difficult grip – like on fingertips only, with limited number of fingers, or with thick bar...)
- ◆ Wrist curls, reverse wrist curls
- ◆ Sledgehammer levering
- ◆ Specialized grip training (hand gripper training, pinch grip training, thick bar training, and endurance grip training – like the farmer's walk or hangs on a pull-up bar)

To devise a workout plan for general overall body strength, you can combine any number of the exercises listed here in a routine that covers all the basic movement patterns and splits them over the course of a whole week (two to six days per week, ideally three to five – one is not enough and seven is too much).

Here are three different examples:

Example 1):

Monday (walking, running, and jumping; climbing):
- Squats
- Front squats
- Pull-ups

Wednesday (throwing; lifting and carrying):
- Military shoulder press
- Bench press
- Deadlifts
- Bent-over rows

Friday (hitting; dexterity):
- Abdominal exercises
- Wrist curls and reverse wrist curls
- Specialized grip training (hand gripper training, pinch grip training, thick bar training)

Note: Biting is skipped because the aspiring athlete has no interest in teeth strength feats and regularly eats raw vegetables, nuts, and dried meat.

Example 2):

Monday (walking, running, and jumping):
- Leg press
- Leg extension
- Leg curl
- Calf raises

Wednesday (throwing; climbing; dexterity 1):
- Bench press
- Military shoulder press
- Triceps extension
- Pull-ups
- Pull-ups on finger tips

Friday (lifting and carrying; dexterity 2; biting):
- ♦ Deadlifts
- ♦ Thick bar deadlifts
- ♦ Farmer's walk
- ♦ Biceps curl
- ♦ Wrestler's bridges

Note: For hitting, the athlete does abdominal exercises each morning.

Example 3):

Monday (walking, running, and jumping; hitting):
- ♦ Sprints
- ♦ Hurdles
- ♦ Sledgehammer swings

Wednesday (throwing; biting):
- ♦ Spear throwing
- ♦ Shot put
- ♦ Wrestler's bridges

Friday (climbing; dexterity):
- ♦ Pull-ups
- ♦ Pull-ups with limited number of fingers
- ♦ Pull-ups on thick bar
- ♦ Pull-ups on finger tips

Saturday (lifting and carrying):
- ♦ Deadlifts
- ♦ Farmers walk

As you can see, I have kept things rather simple, and in actual fact a workout plan for general overall body strength can and should be fairly simple. It is the exercises and the lifting, the sets and repetitions that should be difficult, not the drafting of the plan. The first two workout plans are not unlike basic bodybuilding or powerlifting training. The exercises, and the way they are split over the week, could of course also be grouped according to muscle groups instead of movement patterns. Despite the endless possibilities of combination, the basic exercises for the body are always similar, simply because all human bodies are built according to the same construction plan.

7. Feats of strength: Finding your calling

Now that I have talked a little bit about the many possibilities of training the limited set of human movement patterns, and after I have mentioned the choice you have between turning the training for any of these into specialized training for a feat of strength, or just general training for a balanced development (as in the workout plans above), I want to turn my attention to the question of how to make this difficult choice.

In an earlier section of this book I have talked about the fact that many oldtime strongmen are characterized by their versatility, especially in contrast to the ongoing trend towards specialization in strength sports. Still, I believe that it would be a wise decision to limit oneself somewhat in the choice of oldtime strongman feats one wants to perform or train for. What I mean is simply that it is hard to become great at every feat of strength there is. Therefore, I advise people to find a limited number of feats of strength they want to become truly good at and focus their attention on these.

Also, for true greatness it may be beneficial to limit oneself to only one specific area of expertise, at least temporally (although this can become a source for boredom). I myself tend to be more of a universalist, with the downside of having no area where I am truly *great* at, as I must admit. What I mean is, I have not yet performed a record feat of strength that remains unbeaten, or that, at most, only a handful of people in the world can replicate. My asset is, however, that I have performed several very *diverse* feats of strength that can be considered world-class, in particular for a drug-free athlete, as I am. Thus, I have decided to make the following four different areas my focus:

1. Stone lifting
2. Steel bending, in particular nail and horseshoe bending
3. Grip strength
4. Teeth strength

As this is a very wide array of feats of strength already, one might ask where the specialization lies. However, mind you that I have erased many other possibilities from my list. For example, I do not have a strong ambition any more to become truly great at any of the powerlifting disciplines – the squat, the bench press, and the deadlift. The reasons for this are that there is an extreme competition within these disciplines, because results can too easily be distorted by the use of specialized powerlifting clothing ("equipment") and performance-enhancing drugs. Even in drug tested competitions, the chances of witnessing truly natural performances are nowhere near a hundred per cent. As it has thus become exceedingly difficult to shine with a great performance as a natural athlete (although I do know natural athletes who have won medals at an international level), I have decided to channel my efforts into different directions.

Also, you will notice that I have no overhead shoulder press or push press on my list, although these are classic oldtime strongman feats and although I believe that I have quite a bit of overhead strength to show for. I have at one point managed to lift 100kg (221lbs), my own body weight, in the military shoulder press for several repetitions, and I have once, the first time I tried, cleaned and jerked 130kg (287lbs), without any prior training in the technique of this exercise. Also, it is hardly a challenge for me to push press a dumbbell weighing 70kg (155lbs), and more, one-handedly. However, I leave truly great overhead lifts to the Olympic weightlifters and the modern strongmen, who specialize in such feats, and many of whom, again, have an advantage over me through the use of performance-enhancing drugs (I hate to have to mention this again and again).

Next to the reasons of why I have *not* put some feats on my list, there are, of course, reasons why I *have* put others onto the list. I have put stone lifting on the list, for example, because I have always been a fairly good lifter. Before the age of 18, I could deadlift 252kg (556lbs), with a cheap, inflexible bar and small, rusty plates – having trained at home completely on my own until then. Also, when I travelled to Scotland to lift the Inver Stone and the Dinnie Stones after only a few weeks of specialized training, I was positively surprised how well my attempts went. In particular the Dinnie Stones surprised me as much easier to lift without belt or straps than I had imagined. Further, it did not take much for me to appreciate the idea of lifting a natural stone outdoors, in the clear Highland air, in contrast to all the endless hours of lifting in all these small, cramped gyms in terrible need of a good dusting, which I had come to visit over the years.

That I put steel bending on the list was at first due to necessity, because, when I was preparing for my first performances and looking for feats of strength I could learn quickly, it turned out that steel bending, in particular nail bending, came to me quite easily. It did not take much training for me to be able to bend quite tough nails with the underhand technique, and after a few years of performing regularly, I could bend 230mm (9in) nails with minimal pads, without any apparent effort, and with a smile on my face. At some point sooner or later I considered bending an Ironmind Red Nail, to have some kind of 'official' qualification for being an avid nail bender. Thus, I ordered some blue nails, some red nails, and the original pads from this company. I had realised that most people bend these kinds of nails with the overhand technique, which I had never used before in my nail bending. It took some time for me to really understand the technique, and to understand that it is more of a *pushing* than an actual *bending* motion. However, once I had realized this, after some training with the blue nails, I bent the Red Nail in training the first time I really tried!

Horseshoe bending I found a bit more difficult, but even here it only took me a few months of specialized progressive training, and experimenting with different kinds of leather for pads, until I successfully bent a side-clipped Kerckhaert sx7 horseshoe, size 000, beyond 180 degrees. According to my knowledge, this is an acceptable benchmark in the (small) world of horseshoe bending. Granted, I had regularly bent lighter horseshoes in my shows for years before, which certainly helped, for reasons I will explain in more detail below. However, in sum, it seems that I have a talent for steel bending, although I was never particularly passionate about it and had only started with it because I was in need of a feat for my first strongman shows. By the way, many steel bending feats are wrist strength feats in essence, as the wrist is often the weak link.

Grip strength training is something I should say I am a bit more passionate about, although I neither have the ideal prerequisites for it (I have, for example, rather small hands, making them less suitable for grip strength feats with thick bars), nor have I achieved any outstanding feat of grip strength yet. However, I have done quite well in grip strength competitions, I have lifted the Dinnie Stones without straps (and in my opinion the weak link in this feat is the grip, rather than lifting strength), and have repeatedly closed an Ironmind #3 hand gripper, albeit not with the handles the official width, but only about three centimetres apart. I am also able to deadlift 220kg (486lbs) with four fingers only (index and middle fingers, reverse grip), 140kg (309lbs) with two fingers only (middle fingers, reverse grip), and to lift 90kg (200lbs) on an Ironmind Rolling Thunder deadlift handle. Still, I am far from satisfied with my grip strength and continue to work on it and improve it.

However, I was always interested in grip strength training, even when I was still primarily a bodybuilder in my early youth and a powerlifter after that. As a bodybuilder, for example, I put a special focus on forearm training and pumped out endless repetitions of heavy wrist curls. As a powerlifter, I regularly did simple grip strength exercises to make sure my grip would not be the weak link in my deadlifting. I regularly did, for example, pull-ups on my fingertips, or pull-ups with three, two, or one finger per hand, using two slings of rope to hold onto. Also, I made a point of always using the barbell with the smoothest surface when I did my deadlifting training, instead of a bar with good knurling that would aid my grip. Eventually, my hands would never open up in a deadlift attempt after that.

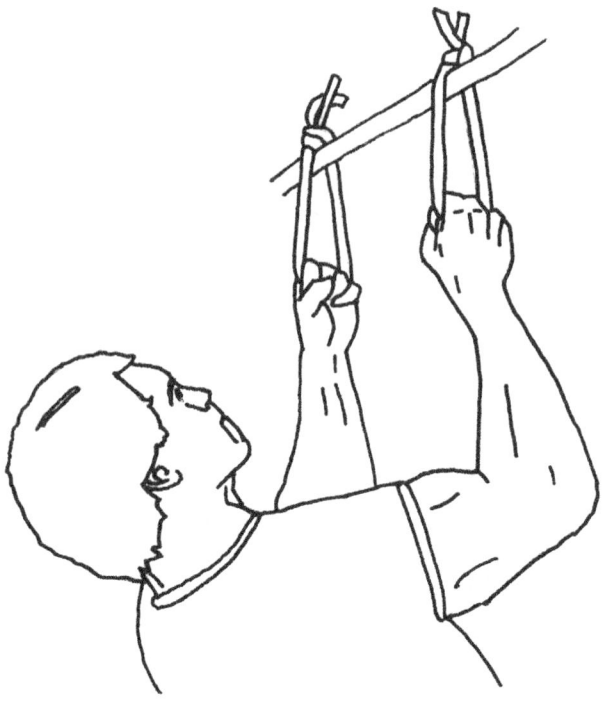

Figure 7.1 Pull-ups on slings of rope.

Teeth strength feats I took up for similar reasons as steel bending. I would never have started with any of these if it had not been for the prospect of doing a strongman show on the street. I had in fact been interested in teeth strength before, having read about such feats in the Guinness Book of World Records as a youth (of course, at that time I was unaware that I would later in my life meet some of the strongmen who had set these records, like Rainer Schröder and Georges Christen!). However, I only developed any real motivation to start training for such feats seriously once I had to put together a strongman show. By then, the choice to try teeth strength feats was obvious, as these are ideal for a *show*: They 1) are seldom seen, they 2) are a bit sensationalist and thrilling, and they 3) are something which everyone can relate to in a way, because everyone in an audience has worried about losing some of their teeth at one point in time, even if only because they bit on some tough piece of food.

In sum, you notice that there may be several criteria by which you can choose your "calling" of the category of strength feat you want to get better or truly great at. Either you choose one category because you are truly passionate about it. Be it for some personal reason, like, for example, one of your ancestors having performed a similar feat. Or, you try lots of different feats and realize that you have some talent for one or the other, making particularly fast progress in it, or achieving world-class level fairly quickly. Or, you choose a particular feat because you *have to*, like I, who had to find feats for a strongman show (although I must say that this is probably a rather unlikely scenario for most people and also not the most pleasant motivation for choosing a training goal).

In any case, I strongly advise you to make some kind of decision like this early on in your career. It is rather hard to become great at lots of different categories of strength feats simultaneously. It is better to focus, at least for some time, or until you have achieved the benchmark you set yourself. You always have the option of taking up another category of strength feat later on. Thus, for example, you might want to start out with grip strength training until you achieve a certain feat, and then change your focus to steel bending and try achieving a different feat there.

8. How to get better at any feat of strength

When amateurs witness a feat of strength, or even have a go at it themselves, they should wonder how it is humanly possible to achieve something like this – this is the purpose of any feat of strength. The truth is that the ability of the strongman to perform the feat is only the result of long years of careful preparation and step-by-step training, and the ability to pursue a goal with patience and perseverance, while overcoming any setbacks along the way. When one tries to do the same, it can become a frustrating experience to reach a plateau and see a goal still out of reach, even after several years of rigorous training. I will be honest with you and say that some goals (in terms of strength, but also in other areas of life) will *never* be reached if the athlete does not have the (genetic or physical) *potential* to reach it. I am not trying to discourage you, I am simply telling you the truth. However, I will try to tell you how you can *increase your chances* to reach any goal in terms of strength training, or in other words, how you can achieve the goals for which you have the theoretical potential.

In general, I believe there are four principles to consider, which I will explain in detail in the following:

1. Progression
2. Continuity
3. Variation
4. Partialisation

When you start with your training for any feat of strength, and when you reach a plateau in your training, you have these four principles to choose from, or to combine, to inspire further improvement. By applying these four principles, you will be able to achieve any feat of strength for which you have the theoretical potential. Let us now have a closer look at them:

1. Progression: This is the simplest and most obvious principle, and always the best to start with. It simply means that any great feat of strength started out as a very little feat of strength. Someone who is able to deadlift 300kg (662lbs) might have started out with 60kg (132lbs) and done nothing else but increase the weight on the bar ever so often. In this example it seems quite obvious, but for some strange reason people do not even consider this possibility in a demonstration of a great feat of strength. Let us assume someone witnesses a teeth lift of only 100kg (221lbs). They might say, "Incredible! If I tried that, the weight would tear out all my teeth at once!" However, just like the 300kg (662lbs) deadlift, the feat seems not impossible at all if you visualize how the strongman started out

by doing teeth lift sets with repetitions of 2.5kg (5.5lbs), then, after some weeks, increased the weight to 5kg (11lbs), and so on. It is really as simple as that.

However, the more abstract a feat of strength becomes, the harder this progression becomes for people to imagine. Let us take the bending of a horseshoe. You cannot increase or reduce the weight on a horseshoe, can you? Yes, but you can always find a horseshoe that is lighter or thinner, or consists of softer steel. You only have to find it, and once you have, and have bent such a horseshoe a hundred times, the next, tougher horseshoe will be within reach.

Or, to look at it from a different perspective: The part of the horseshoe that has to give in when you want to bend it is the very centre of the shoe. So, if this part were weaker or thinner, you would be able to bend it, right? So why not simply make a small cut into the centre, maybe cut halfway through it, and perhaps you will be able to bend a horseshoe that seemed impossible until then. You do this a hundred times, you bend a hundred of these horseshoes with a cut halfway through the centre, you get this kind of practice, and, naturally, your strength increases. Then, the next time you only cut a quarter of the way into the centre of the horseshoe, and, perhaps by now you will be able to bend this as well. And so on.

Or, another possibility: You realize that bending a horseshoe it so tough because it gives you so little leverage. It is a commonly know fact that the smaller a horseshoe is, the harder it becomes to bend, because the leverage decreases. Considering this fact, you could artificially increase the leverage by putting two steel pipes onto the handles. Every once in a while, you use shorter steel pipes as handles, then you do away with one of them completely, and then you discard the other one, and finally you are able to bend the horseshoe without this aid. All of this can take a very long time, of course. Time is a factor that can never be taken out of the equation by natural law.

There is, however, one setback to the principle of progression. It does not work very well with single repetitions. Let us assume you are trying to reach a specific benchmark, like deadlifting 200kg (442lbs). The most obvious way to go about it would probably be to start your first workout with single deadlifts of your current maximum, for example 100kg (221lbs). The next week you try to deadlift 110kg (243lbs) for one repetition, the week after that 120kg (265lbs), and so on:

1st Week: 3 sets of 100kg (221lbs) x 1
2nd Week: 3 sets of 110kg (221lbs) x 1
3rd Week: 3 sets of 120kg (221lbs) x 1

...

In the beginning, especially as a novice, you will certainly have some success. However, from experience I can say that the stronger you become and the more outstanding your aim becomes, the harder it will become for you to continue making gains with this method. Do not ask me about the specific physiological and biological reasons behind this, but it seems that it is much easier to make strength gains with a slightly higher repetition range, with three to six repetitions per set of an exercise, rather than with single repetitions. There are two different methods of doing this you might want to try, both of which work equally well. The first is choosing a specific repetition range you like, not too high and not too low, for example five, but anything between three and six. Then you continue working with sets of this repetition range and make it your aim to slightly increase the resistance of the exercise every once in a while. For example:

1st Week: 3 sets of 90kg (199lbs) x 5
2nd Week: 3 sets of 92.5kg (204lbs) x 5
3rd Week: 3 sets of 92.5kg (204lbs) x 5
4th Week: 3 sets of 95kg (210lbs) x 5
…

Then, after a considerable stint of working with this method, you can try out your maximum in a single repetition again. If you did everything right and if you were able to increase your maximum in five repetitions considerably, your absolute maximum in one repetition will have increased as well. This is probably the best way to train for any feat of strength on a long-term basis.

As a side note, there are those people who tell you that you have to do exactly five sets of five repetitions, then increase the weight next week and do five sets again, no matter how many repetitions you can do, even if you do not manage to do the full five repetitions on every set, for example:

1st set: 5 repetitions
2nd set: 5 repetitions
3rd set: 4 repetitions
4th set: 3 repetitions
5th set 1 repetition

Then you stick with this weight until you achieve the full five by five sets, and after this you increase the weight again.

However, I do not recommend this system, however, which is commonly called the "five by five system" or something of the sort. I find it much too complicated and frustrating, and I find the five sets per exercise tedious. Three sets per exercise are fine. It saves time and allows you to do more exercises in your workout.

The second method you could try, commonly called the pyramid system, works in the following manner: You start with sets of a number of repetitions in the mid-range, for example ten or eight, and with the weight you can lift so many times. Then, every other week or so, you increase the weight considerably and decrease the number of repetitions accordingly. For example:

1st Week: 3 sets of 80kg (177lbs) x 8
2nd Week: 3 sets of 80kg (177lbs) x 8
3rd Week: 3 sets of 90kg (199lbs) x 6
4th Week: 3 sets of 90kg (199lbs) x 6
5th Week: 3 sets of 100kg (221lbs) x 4
6th Week: 3 sets of 100kg (221lbs) x 4

...

In the final week of such a cycle you then try your maximum weight for one repetition. This method works well if you want to work towards a very specific date on which you hope to lift your maximum weight, the best example being a competition on a given day. Of course, you can never tell exactly what your maximum weight on this day will be beforehand, but you can at least set yourself a goal and work towards it. The best example for this system is training for a powerlifting meet, and in fact it is the simplest, most straightforward, and one of the most efficient methods of training for powerlifting. It goes a long way, and most other regimen and workout plans for powerlifting competitions complicate matters unnecessarily.

Until now, what I talked about will already be common knowledge to many advanced trainees, and be quite obvious with regard to, for example, training for the deadlift. The trick is now to adapt these simple schemes for the various oldtime strongman feats. This can be quite a challenge. The schemes work well with feats like the teeth lift or the one-finger lift, and other, related lifts where the weight is simply increased step by step. But let us take stonelifting, for example. It is impossible to find several natural lifting stones with the same shape, but small, consecutive weight differences. I will talk about some particular feats of strength and how to train for them in the next section, but let me emphasize – or rather repeat – here that oldtime strongman training always calls for some creativity, much more than a "simple" weightlifting training where you "only" have to add a weight plate to your bar every once in a while. For example, maybe you can find a way to attach weight plates to a lighter lifting stone with straps, ropes, or chains, and thus increase the weight step by step, as on a weightlifting bar. Or you find a different *kind* of progression instead of increasing the weight, for example the distance you carry a stone, or, even simpler, the duration you can stand upright while holding the stone. Then there is no need for repetitions any more, as the duration of muscle tension of, let us say, walking 20 metres (21 yards) with a stone is already comparable to a set of several repetitions with a regular weight.

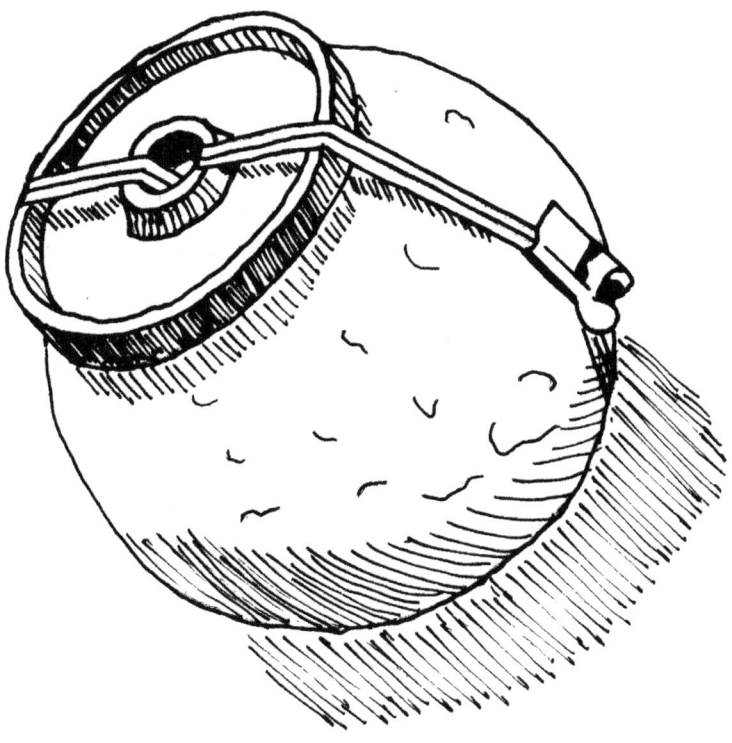

Figure 8.1 Atlas stone with additional weight.

In other cases, however, you will have to find a different approach. Take horseshoe bending again. Bending one horseshoe can be considered one set of one repetition. So is bending five horseshoes in a row, without any break in between each go, one set of five repetitions? Is bending five horseshoes, with a short break in between each go, five sets of one repetition? If I want to do three sets of five repetitions to train for horseshoe bending, do I need fifteen horseshoes per week? This would be quite a costly undertaking. I will talk more about how to train effectively for horseshoe bending below, but the bottom line is that you cannot apply the multiple-repetition approach to any feat of strength easily, and in some cases you will *have to* work with single repetitions. The gist is: adding resistance progressively is one of the key ingredients to achieving any feat of strength. It can turn a seemingly otherworldly feat into something quite achievable.

One further note: The best way to ensure you stick to the principle of progression is to use a very simple tool during your workouts – pen and paper. All you have to do is note down the exercises of your current training plan, and the maximum weight you have lifted in the last workout (and the number of repetitions you have performed with it). The next time you do the same exercise, you review what you have lifted last time and try to outperform it. If you are able to lift more weight for the same number of repetitions, or do more repetitions with the same weight, you have progression. Then you can cross out the numbers from last time and write the new numbers down. It is no problem if you are *not* able to outperform your last performance each time – it is a complete misconception to believe you can make progress on each exercise every week. However, keep an eye on it and see if you can make progress some other week.

This is really the simplest way to keep track of your progress, and it is highly effective. It can mean the one difference between an athlete who excels in gaining great strength, and one who fails to do so: One of them had pen and paper in his pocket, whereas the other had not. Do not make the mistake of believing that you can memorize all the weights you lifted on all the exercises you did in a certain week. It is one of the things that are most easily forgotten. I have been training with weights for more than twenty years now and keep forgetting how much I lifted on a certain day the minute I walk out of the gym door.

2. Continuity: Much of what I just said seems obvious and simple. In truth, matters *are* quite simple in oldtime strongman training, at least with regard to putting a workout plan together. The harder part is obviously to stick to it and to manage to make that progression in all those little steps. Therefore, continuity is another principle an aspiring oldtime strongman has to pay attention to, in particular as some oldtime strongman feats require long periods of training until they are achieved. Any of the methods described above and below, like progressively adding resistance, is useless if not stuck to for weeks, months, or years, depending on how much out of reach the feat of strength yet is. In some cases, this obviously requires patience, but there is no remedy to this. As I mentioned before, time is a factor that cannot be taken out of the equation, because biology dictates that muscles and tendons take a certain time to develop, grow, and become stronger. At the same time, your nervous system needs to learn a new movement, like a lifting or bending technique, and this takes time as

well – an aspect that must not be disregarded, and which I will talk about in more detail below. In sum, train the exercise or feat regularly. Start with a resistance you can manage, but increase the resistance ever so often. Do this continuously, week by week, and month by month, and, in small steps, you will get closer to your aim. It is actually this simple.

3. Variation: However, even a trainee who sticks to these first two principles rigorously will hit a wall every now and then and reach a plateau. No matter how hard he tries, he will not be able to lift more than, say, 100kg (221lbs) for 5 repetitions. Since several weeks or even months, every time he tries to put even 101.25kg (223.5lbs) on his lifting device, he is only able to do four repetitions. Then the trainee will have to resort to another key principle, which is variation. This is to be understood in two ways: a) variation to introduce new training stimuli, and b) variation to refine the technique.

Let us talk about a) first. You might have already heard or read about how bodybuilders typically train. They constantly try to find new ways to train a certain muscle or muscle group – new exercises, new variations of an exercise, a new grip variation on a certain exercise, new angles, stances, and so on. For example, a serious bodybuilder will not only do pull-ups with a regular, shoulder-width overhand grip, but he will do this for several weeks, then switch to a very wide grip for some weeks, then to a parallel grip, and then to a very close underhand grip, and so on. He will train his back and arm muscles from a great variety of angles and with a great variety of exercises, because he hopes that this kind of *variation* will constantly confuse his muscles and create new impulses for them to adapt and grow. The principle is comparable to progressive resistance, which is also meant to constantly pose a challenge to your body that your muscles have to adapt to, and it actually works.

A strongman will have to do something similar if he wants to increase his chances of gaining oldtime strength, but in a slightly adapted way. Let us assume you are training for a grip strength feat, like lifting a certain weight on a thick handled barbell. You are already progressively increasing resistance, adding weights plates to the bar in small, consecutive steps. You also do this continuously, obediently sticking to your workout plan of training for this feat every Friday. Then, you can further increase your chances of reaching your aim by introducing variation to your scheme. However, I would not do this in the way a bodybuilder does it, for example, by varying the width of your grip (although you can do this as well in principle, see below), but I would understand it as adding different grip strength exercises to your workout plan to *complement* this kind of thick bar grip strength training. For example, you add some pinch grip exercises and some hand gripper training to your workout plan. Even if you have no ambition to reach a particular goal with these exercises, the training of your grip with a variety of slightly different movements will train your gripping muscles from lots of different angles. This will increase your potential in the same monotonous thick handled barbell lifting exercise as well.

Or, to take another example, stone lifting: Let us assume you have found your lifting stone for training, and a way of progressively adding resistance. Then it will help you to do a variety of other lifting exercises, like stiff-legged deadlifts and bent-over rows, because then you have some variety in your training. What I practically mean is, you maintain continuity in training your one feat of strength, and add variety by doing a number of additional, complementary exercises. You can then also introduce more variety within these additional exercises, for example, varying grip-width when doing stiff-legged deadlifts, as in the last example.

In addition to this kind of variation, you can experiment with b) varying your technique, especially when you get stuck or reach a plateau. It is quite often the case than one is in very close reach of achieving a certain feat of strength, and longing to bridge this last gap. But the very last step is often the hardest! Varying your technique in the training for the feat of strength is another possibility you can try here. Let us take the example of the thick barbell lift again and let us assume your aim is to lift 180kg (397lbs) on this bar, but get stuck at a best of 160kg (353lbs). You cannot seem to make any further progress, although you firmly believe that you have the potential to lift 180kg (397lbs). What you could try then is, for example, if you have used the conventional deadlifting technique so far, to switch to a sumo deadlifting technique for a change. Or, you try a slightly different grip, for example a thumbless grip. Or, you try not to curl your forearms at the beginning of the movement, and so on.

Let us take nail bending as a different example. Since several months, you simply do not manage to bend the one nail you aim at. Then, try a different sort of padding, or roll it up more tightly, or try a different sort of leather, or try to place the nail differently in your hand, and so on. Most of these experiments will probably lead you nowhere and make the feat even harder. However, there is a chance that one of these variants will actually be the small improvement or change you needed to get over the wall you hit.

4. Partialisation: Some feats of strength have it in their nature that they represent a complex movement and are therefore particularly difficult to train, or, as mentioned above, particularly difficult to train with several repetitions. In this case (but also in many other cases), it can help to analyse the feat of strength, break it down into parts, and train these parts separately, or some of these parts in addition to the training of the com-

plete feat of strength. If you look at horseshoe bending, for example, you realize that the feat consists of several phases: a) the first kink, which is usually the hardest part psychologically, then b) the phase which some people call the sweep, which is the actual 'opening up' of the horseshoe. Then you change your grip on the object, readjust your thigh padding (if you are using one), brace the centre of the shoe against your thigh (close to your hip, as in bending a regular steel bar on your thigh), and c) finish the bend by pushing down on the 'handles' of the horseshoe. By then you have bent the horseshoe into an S-shape, and this is where the feat stops if it is one of your harder horseshoes. With a lighter horseshoe, you could go on to d) bending it into a heart-shape between your thighs.

Thus, the different phases of the bend require different muscles and muscle groups. Phase a) and b) require great grip strength, as well as some pulling strength in the one arm, some pushing strength in the other arm, and quite a bit of forearm strength in both arms (the kind of strength you would require to lever a sledgehammer in front of your body). Phase c) requires mostly pushing strength from both arms (chest and triceps) and from your abdomen, as well as some of the forearm strength just described, and some pain tolerance and isometric tension in your thigh. Phase d), if there is one, requires some chest strength and strength from your hip adductors.

With this kind of knowledge you have different options of what I call *partialisation* in your training. You can, for example, train the involved body parts separately, with exercises like the bench press, hand gripper training, and sledgehammer levering, either *instead of*, or *in addition to*, your horseshoe bending training. Or, if you realize that one of these phases is a particular weakness of yours, you can put a special emphasis on this phase for some time, for example phase c), which you could improve on with simple braced steel bar bending, for example. Or you "pre-bend" some horseshoes with the help of a vice, so that you can train this phase separately, without even having to do phase b) and c).

To conclude, these four principles, when applied in training, make a seemingly unattainable feat of strength attainable. I have listed them here in an order of importance, i.e. the principles of progression and continuity are the most important ones, which must be observed by all means. Following these, the principles of variation and partialisation are optional, but they are basic tools that can lead to further progress.

9. Some popular feats of strength and how to train for them, or: How to make progress on a specific feat of strength

Now that I have talked a little bit about general principles for the mastery of oldtime strongman feats, also by giving a few examples, I want to focus in more detail on specific feats of strength and how to train for them. As you will certainly know, there is a great variety of oldtime strongman feats, although some of these are, granted, only variations of a few basic (categories of) feats. As there are several books available that demonstrate this great variety (my favourite being Charles MacMahon's *Feats of Strength and Dexterity*), I want to take a different approach: I will pick only a few popular categories of oldtime strongman feats I have mastered well so far, and cover these in a bit more detail to tell you how I trained for them.

As a disclaimer, I should probably mention that there have also been whole books covering the one or the other of these feats, obviously in more detail than I can do here, for reasons of space.

I should also mention again that I started out as a bodybuilder, with a regular focus on strength training, and after this trained as a powerlifter for several years before I even took up oldtime strongman training. Thus, I already had a considerable level of strength when I started out with training for any of the following feats. This you should take into consideration, as it is obviously harder to start out with feats of strength from nought, without any prior experience in strength sports whatsoever.

And as a last comment before I begin this section, I should also tell you a little bit about my general attitude towards training for feats of strength. My approach is very focused and work-oriented. As I make (part of) a living out of being an oldtime strongman, my attitude towards certain feats of strength is almost *dispassionate* when compared to other trainees. I work on the feats of strength of my choice to either a) make them part of my show, or b) to achieve a certain benchmark to strengthen my reputation, i.e. to demonstrate that I am also strong in real life, and that I am qualified to step on a stage and do a strength demonstration. I do so mostly by focusing on one feat at a time, until I have either mastered it, or until another feat becomes more important. Thus, I do not have the kind of passionate, spiritual, or esoteric relationship to certain feats of strength that others have.

Furthermore, I look at my training as working hours, not much different from going to an office to do a job. I do obviously enjoy this "job" a lot, but I still consider it something that simply needs to be done.

I believe that this kind of attitude is a good thing. It has helped me a lot to achieve different feats of strength without emotions getting in my way. Also, if you do not perceive your training as your one and only life-defining aspect, you become much less frustrated when your training is not going so well. I am not trying to say that my way is the only way, or the only way that works. Quite the contrary, I admire those people who go about their training with a great amount of passion and spiritual inspiration – but my approach is systematic, straightforward, and technical, rather than emotional.

In the following, I want to talk about seven categories, or disciplines, of strength feats and how to train for them:

1. Natural stonelifting
2. Harness lifting
3. Nail bending
4. Horseshoe bending
5. Grip strength feats
6. Teeth strength
7. (Kettlebell) juggling

9.1. Natural stonelifting

The first discipline I want to talk about is natural stonelifting, as this is such an atavistic type of feat. In principle, people might have practised stonelifting since the Palaeolithic (the *Stone* Age), although we only have proof for it since Greek antiquity. I emphasize the "natural" in stonelifting to make clear that I am talking about stones that nature has shaped, in contrast to the so-called Atlas stones, which have an almost perfect spherical shape, are usually made of concrete, and belong into the field of modern strongman sports. Although Atlas stone lifting is popular with audiences and visually impressive as well, it lacks some of the poetry and minimalism of lifting a natural stone. This being said, there are also natural stones nearing a spherical shape – the most famous one being the Inver Stone, about which I will talk more below.

Although lifting a heavy natural stone is such a simple and basic feat of strength, and so beautiful to watch (if not done by an uncouth and obnoxious lifter), I have seen it performed rather seldom in stage performances. This might be so because a heavy stone is rather uncomfortable to transport from one show location to the next. Anton von Kaltenberg, a German performing strongman of recent times, has regularly performed it at the *Kaltenberger Ritterturnier*, one of the largest medieval festivals in Europe, taking place every summer in Bavaria. His stonelifting feat was always a highlight and very popular with audiences.

The big question with natural stonelifting training is always the goal of the trainee. As there is no linear progression in terms of kilograms or pounds, no stones that are exactly the same shape but different in weight, there is no "benchmark" to reach, in arbitrary terms. Rather, benchmarks in stonelifting are specific, commonly known stones, famous for being a great challenge to lift. Thus, one aim in stonelifting training could be a) to lift one of these famous stones. However, a different goal could be b) lifting a big natural stone you came across by chance (although it is not world-famous), for example, to regularly lift it in a strongman stage performance. In this case, the stone obviously needs to be sufficiently heavy to lift, not just for you to justify stepping on a stage and calling yourself a strongman, but also to make sure regular guys from the street will not replicate the feat easily. A third goal could be simply c) training with stones to gain general strength, to toughen yourself up, to spend time outdoors, and to save money on training equipment – in short, as a means to an end. However, I only want to talk about a) here as an example, because the methods and principles of training for the famous and well-known stones apply to b) and c) as well.

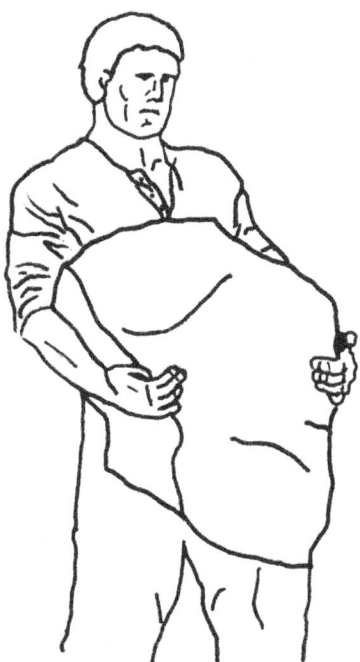

Figure 9.1 Natural stonelifting.

How to lift a famous and well-known stone: The first thing you should do with any famous stone you want to lift, is to gather some data and information on the stone: its exact weight (obviously), its rough measurements, its properties (does it have a rough surface or is it rather slippery), and what the specific challenge connected to this stone actually is (to lift it once, to lift it to a certain height, or to carry it, for example). From this you can usually conclude what kinds of muscle groups and exact movements are needed to do the lift, and what constitutes the weak link. Following this analysis, you should apply the principles of progression, continuity, variation, and partialisation I described above, to develop a workout plan and train with it over time.

There are not that many really well-known lifting stones in the world. The most famous ones today are probably the Inver Stone (Scotland), the Dinnie Stones (Scotland), and the Husafell Stone (Iceland). As you can see, stonelifting has a tradition in Northern European countries, and there are whole books about the many other not so well-known stones in this area. Different forms of stonelifting are popular in many different cultures around the globe, including the Basque country, Bavaria, and Japan, but as there are not many stones that have reached the kind of international prominence of the three above, I will use those as examples here.

How I trained to lift and shoulder the Inver Stone: The Inver Stone, as I mentioned above, is an almost spherical stone, just slightly egg-shaped, with a relatively smooth surface, although somewhat grainy. All of this can be deducted easily from looking at photographs and films of other people lifting it. The Inver Stone weighs roughly 122kg (268lbs). The challenge is to either lift it to hip-height, to chest-height, to shoulder it, to shoulder it and hold it with one hand only, or to lift it overhead. The feat becomes heavier in this order, but even lifting it to hip-height is a commendable achievement. You are meant to lift the Inver Stone without the help of tacky, but chalk is allowed. Obviously, it is much more difficult to lift when wet, which can happen easily, as the stone is stored outdoors in Great Britain.

You need a strong back and lifting abilities to lift the Inver Stone to hip height, like in a deadlift. Mind you that your back will probably be arched when you deadlift it, which puts great stress on your spine and can be harmful to your lower back. You want to be prepared for rounded-back lifting. Next, you will need an even stronger back to "roll" it to chest height, and then to shoulder height, in a motion not unlike a barbell clean. Here you will also need a strong chest and arms to hold the stone in a "hugging" manner. You will then need a strong core to balance it on your shoulder. If you plan to lift it overhead (only few men achieve this), you will need a tremendous amount of overhead pressing strength. However, the weak link is always your wrist and finger strength, in particular at the beginning of the lift, because the stone is so difficult to hold on to.

Now we have already undertaken a sort of *partialisation*. If you want to train for the Inver Stone with regular training equipment, you should do deadlifts, bent over rows, cleans, core training, barbell flies, biceps curls, wrist curls, grip training (the best variety probably being lifts with a thick bar), bench press, military shoulder press, and the push press. On all of these exercises it is possible to progressively add weight, by simply adding weight plates to the barbells and dumbbells. It might be a good idea to stick with such a training routine for some time until you have built considerable strength and can lift respectable weights in these exercises before you even think of travelling to Scotland.

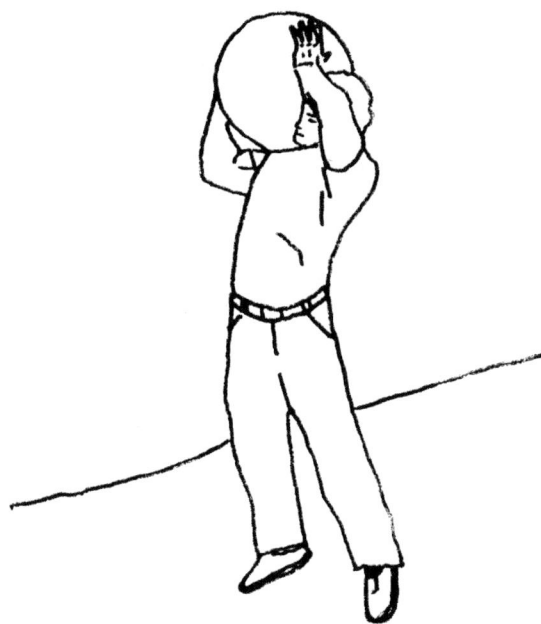

Figure 9.2 Shouldering the Inver Stone.

Once you believe that you have reached such a level, I would strongly recommend that you perform a more specialized training as well, that is, lifting a stone that is close in size, weight, and shape to the Inver Stone. Or, rather, two stones: one that is a bit lighter than the Inver Stone, and one that it similar in weight or even heavier. To find such stones you will obviously have to invest some time and effort searching riverbeds, for example (round stones are typically shaped by water). You will also need a scale to weigh the stone, a vehicle to transport it, and, probably, some assistance to load it. If you only care to gather one training stone, I would strongly recommend that you go for one that is lighter than your challenge stone (in this case the Inver Stone), because you can do a lot more with it, like repetitions. A stone that is heavier or similarly heavy as your challenge stone only serves for a one-repetition maximum attempt.

I had two tools at my disposal to train for the Inver Stone: a) A natural stone I found in a quarry, with a very rough and irregular shape, not round and shaped by water, but tending towards a cuboid shape. It weighed around 105kg (232lbs). b) I had a so-called Atlas stone I had cast myself out of concrete, although this was more of an experiment gone wrong. It had a rather craggy surface, compared to the smooth surface of professional Atlas stones. Also, something had gone wrong with the cast and the stone had a flat bottom, as if someone had cut off the lowest part of it. However, apart from this it had an almost spherical shape and was almost equal in weight to the actual Inver Stone, weighing around 120kg (265lbs). It was less dense, though, and therefore larger.

I started training for the Inver Stone shortly after I had made plans to travel to Scotland to lift the Dinnie Stones. I thought I might want to try this as well while I am there, although I was much more interested in the Dinnie Stones. I performed a stonelifting training twice a week, training for both the Dinnie and the Inver Stone, but with a much greater focus on the former (I will talk about this below).

What I did in terms of specialized training for the Inver Stone was not more than the following: On Tuesdays I would train with the natural lifting stone. This stone was relatively easy to grip and lift to hip-level, like in a deadlift, so I did a couple of sets of this with repetitions to start out with. Here I had a simple possibility for progression, as I could increase the number of repetitions gradually over the weeks. After this, I would try to shoulder the stone, in which I failed the first time I tried, but eventually I could do it for a few repetitions. This was all I did on Tuesdays.

On Thursdays I would train with the Atlas stone. All I would do here were a couple of sets of lifting the stone onto my lap before dropping it again (onto a couple of car tires to make sure it would not break). Here I must admit that I trained with single, maximum repetitions, which I do not principally recommend if you can avoid it, but in this case I did not have much patience with training for the Inver Stone. After eventually realizing that I could lift the 120kg (265lbs) Atlas stone without any troubles, I increased its weight by fixing weight plates to it with a ratchet strap. Thus, I simply increased my maximum weight, until I could lift almost 140kg (309lbs) to hip-level – obviously slightly heavier than the Inver

Stone. I had made the earlier experience that this kind of overcompensation in a specific part of a lift or feat is quite efficient (I had done something similar with lockout-training for powerlifting exercises, for example). And in this manner I had progression on Thursdays as well.

This is all I did for a couple of weeks (I had to book an early flight, so I did not have many weeks to train for the Scottish stones), and I was positively surprised and very happy when I managed to lift and shoulder the Inver Stone on 26 July 2013. During these weeks of preparation I did very little additional training for other muscle groups (NB stonelifting is in principle a great workout for the whole body). Thus, I had applied all the important principles: progression, continuity, variation, and partialisation. I had progression by increasing the number of repetitions on the lighter natural stone and by increasing the weight on the Atlas stone. I had continuity, because I trained two times per week in all the weeks I had left until my journey began (although it would have been wise to schedule some more time). I had variation, as I had two kinds of stones for training, which were very different in shape and demand. And I had partialisation: I trained the initial, (dead)lifting phase with the Atlas stone, emphasising maximum lifts by applying the principle of overcompensation, and I trained the shouldering part with the lighter stone. Both workouts, by the way, were also suitable to increase my pain tolerance, as both stones scraped my skin when I lifted them. Pain tolerance plays an important role in stone lifting.

How I trained to lift the Dinnie Stones: To train for the Dinnie Stones, I split the training for the specific grip strength and the training for the deadlift strength. The first thing I did was to ask my welder to produce two Dinnie-Ring replicas for me. I did not know the exact measurements, but settled for two identical rings with an outer diameter of 18cm (7in) and a thickness of 16mm (0.6in). As it turned out, the original ring on the smaller stone was a little bit smaller, and the original ring on the larger stone was a little bit larger. This made them easier to lift than I had thought.

I then trained my grip for the feat in a very straightforward manner: I simply worked my way up with alternating one-handed deadlifts with one replica ring and a loading pin. All I did was about five single sets per hand, with about three minutes rest in between, and increasing the weight on each attempt and each week. I reserved one day per week for this training only. To toughen my hands additionally, I would do three to five sets of as many pull-ups as I could on the replica rings on a separate day.

Also on a separate day, I would train the specific deadlift strength for this feat. I am naturally strong when it comes to top position deadlifts in a rack, so-called lockout-training, but the fact that you have to lift the stones with one hand in front, and one hand behind your body, calls for special attention. I thus tried to duplicate the situation as closely as I could: I slid the two ring replicas onto a barbell, which I loaded unevenly with weight (to simulate the feeling of having to lift two stones with a different weight). Then I would straddle the bar and work my way up until I could do three repetitions with 330kg (728lbs) on the last training day before my plane left for Scotland. I would usually do two to three warm-up sets and then three working sets, increasing the weight each time and reducing the numbers of repetitions, for example, 5-4-3. However, for this deadlift training I used lifting straps (as I trained my grip on the separate day).

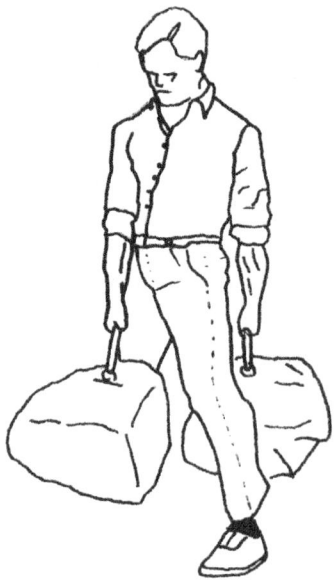

Figure 9.3 Lifting the Dinnie Stones.

I believe these two examples suffice to explain how one can approach stonelifting training to lift a specific, well-known stone. They are only two of endless possibilities, but the take-home message is that it is up to you to find a method that works for you, using creative thinking and the principles of progression, continuity, variation, and partialisation. I do not want to talk much about the Husafell Stone here, as I have never attempted lift it, but if I were to train for lifting and perhaps carrying this stone, I would first try to gather as much information on its dimensions and measurements as I could. Then I would probably use a similar method of training the lifting part with a very heavy stone, and the carrying part with a lighter stone. The latter I would eventually attempt to carry further in training than the Husafell Stone is to be carried, thus overcompensating without taxing my body too much. This being said, I believe that of these three famous stones, the Husafell Stone is the hardest to conquer and requires a very large and heavy athlete who provides sufficient counter-weight to this massive boulder.

9.2. Harness lifting

The harness lift was devised several hundred years ago with the aim of lifting the largest humanly possible weight off the floor – a status for which it contests with the back lift. A harness lift, with a proper harness and a sturdy platform, allows you to activate thighs, gluteus, back, and trapezius to a maximum level, and in the version where the lifter also has parallel bars to hold onto, you can also bring chest and triceps strength into play. Considering that the weight must only be minimally lifted off the floor for the lift to be technically successful (but not necessarily satisfying to an observing audience), these aspects in unison – the strongest muscle groups in your lower body, in combination with some of the strongest muscle groups in your upper body, activated for a minimum range of motion – allow you to lift tremendous weights in a harness lift. Lifting a ton in this manner is nothing unusual, and this has obviously been amply used for show purposes over the centuries. You can theoretically lift horses, oxen, small cars, or a group of humans with a harness, to the great amazement of an audience.

Several years ago, the so-called USAWA, the United States All-Round Weightlifting Association, which trains and tests oldtime strength exercises, has started to perform the harness lift in a sportive manner. They want to determine the exact weights their athletes can lift under competitive circumstances, with standardised rules and equipment. This obviously takes away some of the magic of this feat in comparison to its use for performance purposes, but this is the spirit of our modern times. At present, people are interested in concrete numbers and facts, rather than tales and myths, which is justifiable to a certain degree.

I have only once, just for the fun of it, somewhat tested my limits in the harness lift in training, and managed to lift 900kg (1987lbs). However, in all modesty, I should note that this was not my physical limit, but the limit dictated by the weights I had at hand to load my lifting platform.

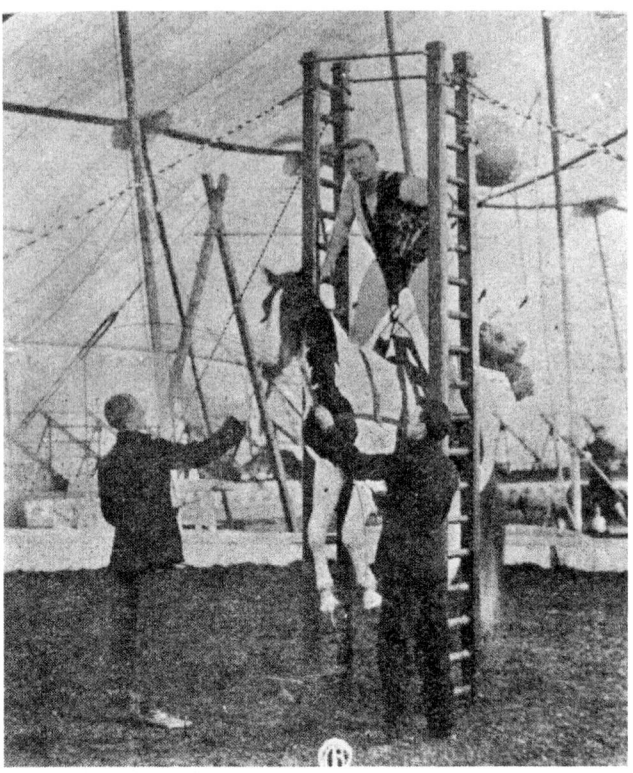

Figure 9.4 With a harness, a strong man can theoretically lift a horse (circus strongman in Brisbane, 1903).

This already brings us to a very important aspect in the harness lift: the equipment. There is no company in the world that constructs lifting harnesses, so you will have to custom-make your own, which is still fairly easy to do. However, the next challenge is to find so much weight and attach it to your harness to lift it safely. Considering these aspects, you will soon realize that the greater challenge in the harness lift lies in finding the right equipment, rather than in doing the actual lift.

I have constructed my harness based on a model of the USAWA, and I am indebted to them for their input and a sketch drawing they provided me with. I do not want to share their ideas here and sell them as my own, so if you want concrete advice on how to make your own harness, I would like to forward you to this association and advise you to contact these friendly gentlemen directly.

My lifting platform is loosely based on historical models, derived from old photographs, and designed to be transportable. I constructed it myself out of old wooden roof beams, with the generous help of my mentor, the acrobat Walter Moshammer, who is also a skilled carpenter and constructs all of his props himself.

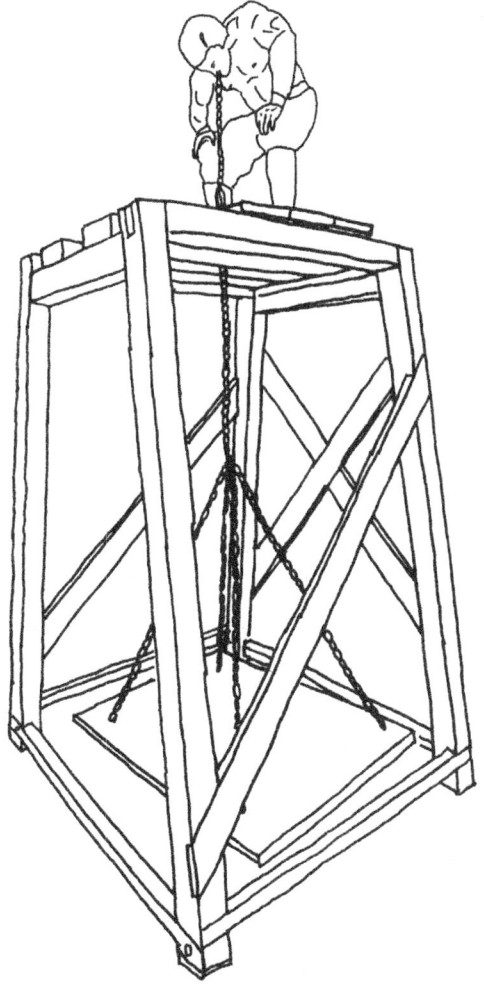

Figure 9.5 My self-made lifting platform (here used for a teeth lift).

Once you have found your harness and a way to attach weight to it, and if you have strong legs, a strong back, and some strength in your triceps and chest, you will very soon be able to lift more than the world record in the deadlift easily. This being said, the question remains how much sense it makes to actually train for the harness lift itself if you do not want to use it for show purposes. And even then, you will probably not need to train with high intensity. I use the harness lift to great effect in my shows since ten years, but I never actually train for it and have never *truly* tested my potential – never going beyond the 900kg (1987lbs) I talked about above.

In my shows, I simply load my lifting platform with children from the audience, and the limit in how much I can lift in this manner is always dictated by the space on the platform and safety considerations, rather than my strength. Nevertheless, the feat is very inspiring to children who witness it, or even participate in it. When a man lifts more than ten children at once, this is a very concrete achievement that children can relate to, memorize, and be inspired by, even if it is no "superhuman" achievement in actual fact.

Also, if children participate in it, and gather up the courage to step onto the platform, the feeling of being hoisted into the air with so many other children at once creates a very "real" sensation of the strongman's strength, when compared to, for example, an athlete simply lifting a heavy barbell. This is only the case, of course, if they are children who have not yet lost their potential for real-life inspiration and fascination, as many grown-ups sadly have.

By the way, this is, in my view, also one of the tasks of an oldtime strongman in our present time: not just to be the strongest and to display this in an arrogant manner, but to be an honest and well-meaning inspiration, and a positive role model to an (especially young) audience. If there is only one life in your audience you can turn around, it is well worth the effort.

I have now digressed somewhat from my topic and want to conclude it by adding that a maximum harness lift is a great stress on the body. It compresses your spine to a considerable degree. It should therefore not be trained regularly with near-maximum weight. Instead, I would train basic lifts like the deadlift, squat, and dips, or bench or shoulder press regularly, to build the muscle groups you need in a harness lift. If you want, you can train partial lifts in all of these movements as well, with lockout exercises. I am a great believer in the effectiveness of such. Then, if you do have a sturdy harness and platform, you can do a maximum attempt in the harness lift now and then, or use it for show purposes, keeping the safety aspect in mind at all times. After a maximum attempt in a harness lift, I recommend you do some pull-ups to stretch your spine a little.

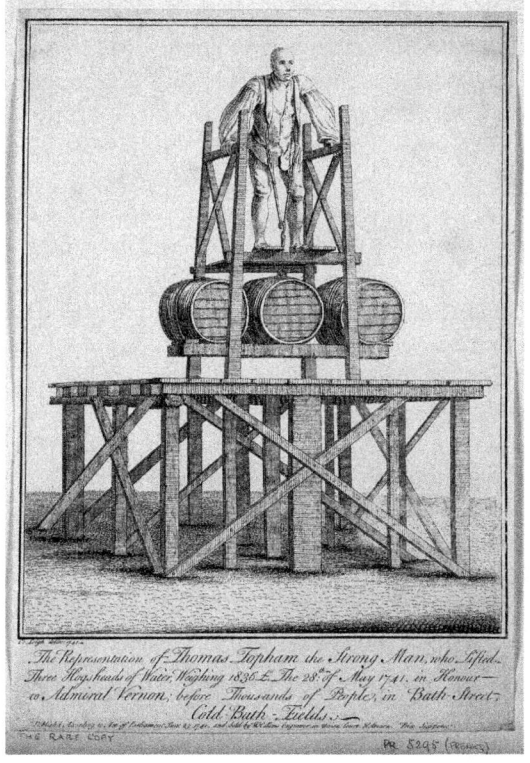

Figure 9.6 Eighteenth-century engraving of British strongman Thomas Topham performing a harness lift. One of the historical models on which I based my lifting platform.

9.3. Nail bending

Nail bending is popular, because nails are easy to get and hard to bend. They are small and can be carried anywhere without effort. Even in our modern world, where less and less people work with their hands, a nail is still an object most people can relate to, as everyone has held a nail in their hands at least once in their life. Also, nail bending has received more attention lately, as standardized "nails" are now being produced and sold to define concrete benchmarks and provide measurable challenges for avid nail benders.

Of course, these are not actual nails, but short steel bars with similar dimensions as nails. They lack a point and a head, and are therefore useless for any other purpose than being bent, which is compensated by a relatively high purchasing price. One should mention here in particular the Ironmind Red Nail, which most avid nail benders want to bend under regulated conditions sooner or later (I did so in 2015), and the Ironmind Gold Nail, which nobody has yet bent under official rules at the moment I am writing this. Because of the increasing popularity of nail bending, I do not want to talk too much about it here, because dozens of instructions on this feat exist by now. However, I will talk a little bit about how I trained to bend large spikes for my shows and how I trained to bend the Red Nail.

I have already explained above how I took up oldtime strongman training out of the necessity of having to perform a show act in front of audiences. One of the first feats I started training for was nail bending, and in the beginning I exclusively used the "underhand" bending technique. The underhand technique is one of two popular bending methods, the other one being the "overhand" technique.

In the underhand technique you grab the nail as in the final position of a pull-up with an underhand grip, that is, with your palms facing your chest. Your hands can be close together or at the very ends of the nail, so that the ends of the nail protrude only very little from your closed hands, and rest about where the thumb separates from the hand. Then you pull down, towards your hip, in the hope of bending the nail to at least 135 degrees. In this phase, your wrist strength is the weak link, but also your grip strength will be greatly challenged.

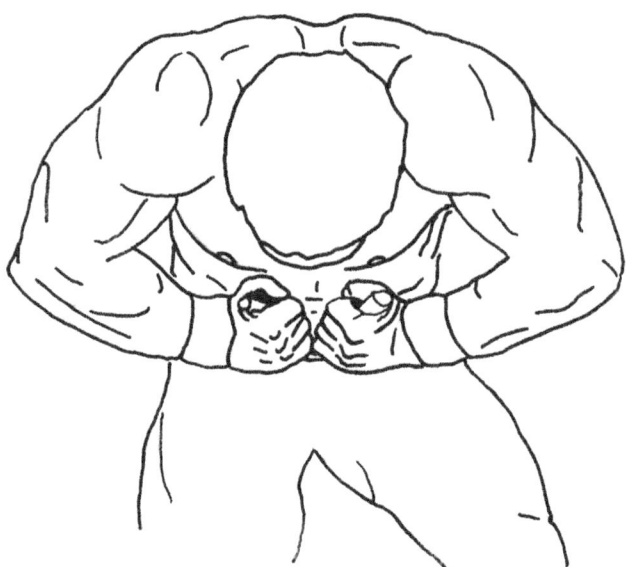

Figure 9.7 Nail bending with the underhand technique.

Once you have bent the nail in this manner, the rest is relatively easy, as you now have to turn it around, with the bent end facing to the ceiling, grab the ends of the nail, and push them together in front of your chest (using chest strength). Here you might want to adjust your hands again towards the end, so that you do not crush your own fingers, but you will do this instinctively.

Once the ends of the nail are about parallel to each other, the bend can be considered complete. However, this is an arbitrary rule. The famous Luxembourgian oldtime strongman Georges Christen, one of the pioneers of recovering the art of oldtime strongman feats after World War II (inspired by the Luxembourgian legend John Grün), set his official world record in nail bending (368 nails bent within 60 minutes) by bending them to about 45 degrees.

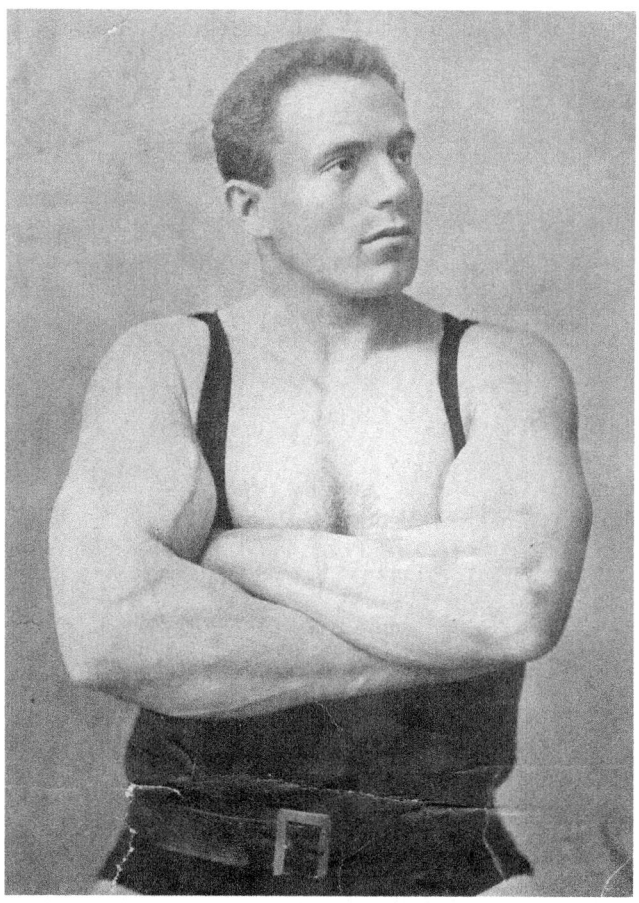

Figure 9.8 John Grün.

Very important in any nail bending are the so-called pads or wraps, which, traditionally, consist of two pieces of leather or cloth you wrap around the ends of the nail, or one piece of cloth you wrap around the whole nail. It has the obvious purpose of protecting your hands from injury. This is important in the underhand technique, but essential in the overhand technique. People have successfully bent nails with all sorts of pads of artificial material, but I would go with leather first, as it is a traditional, natural material, and cheap to get in the small quantities you need for nail bending – perhaps even for free. It does wear out in time, so be cautious and check your leather pads before you bend.

The overhand technique is popular especially with those who bend the modern, standardized "nails" produced by companies like Ironmind. As mentioned above, these are not really nails, but simply short steel bars, and do not have a sharp point. For this reason, the overhand technique can be applied here to make the feat much more achievable. In the overhand technique, you grab the nail, or bar, with an overhand grip in such a manner that the ends rest right in the *centres* of your palms. Here you will already realize that the overhand technique gives you considerably more leverage, because your hands are farther apart. You will also realize how essential pads are for the overhand technique. Otherwise you would push the nails into your palms and pierce your skin. Moreover, you need pads of the sturdiest material possible and they needs to be wrapped around the nail very tightly, because they constitute artificial elongations of the short steel bar that increase the leverage!

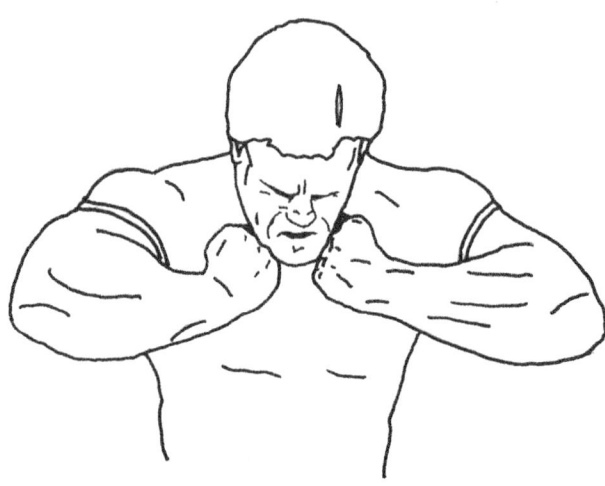

Figure 9.9 Nail bending with the overhand technique.

The bending technique is the following: You start by lifting the nail up to your very throat, that is, the highest position from which you can start, and you lift your elbows up and back as far as you can. Then, with a surge of power, you actually *push* right *into* the ends of the nail. It helps if you imagine that you need to squeeze the nail together, like an accordion, rather than *bend* it. In this manner, you still need a large amount of grip and wrist strength (albeit the opposite strength as for the underhand technique), but arguably the greatest amount of the force that bends the nail initially comes from the chest and shoulder muscles. Also, flexibility is an important factor, as you have an advantage if you are able to lift your elbows high up and far back, so that you can fully exert this power from the chest and shoulders. Once you have thus bent the nail to about 135 degrees, you finish the bend in a similar manner as in the underhand technique, which again requires chest and grip strength.

There is also a third technique to start a nail bend. It is done by holding the nail upright in one hand (let us say, the left hand) in front of your body, near your core, at around hip-level, and then grabbing the upper end of the nail with your other hand (in this case the right hand) with your thumb facing downwards and the tip of your thumb facing towards your body, so that both of the thumbs of your hands are near the centre of the nail. Then you pull down and back with your right hand, that is, towards your body, while your left hand simply tries to hold against this force. Your elbows will automatically move closer together as you exert full strength, and your hands will move away from your body.

Bending, or kinking, a nail in this manner is very impressive visually, much more so than the two techniques described above, but it is also the weakest technique. Therefore, you can try it now and then in your training, but I would really not spend too much time on it. The other two techniques will allow you to bend much harder steel and tougher nails. In this third technique, the final moves are the same as in the underhand and overhand technique.

In fact, finishing any nail bend is always done in a similar manner and always the easier part (if done right away, as long as the steel is still warm). The greatest difficulty always lies in the initial bend, or the kink, as some people say. In theory, there is a fourth technique to get this kink done. It is the easiest and most intuitive one of all: resting the centre of the nail on your thigh, near the hip, and pushing down on the ends of the nail with your hands. This type of bending, which is mostly done with longer steel bars, is generally grouped under "braced bending", which means that you *brace* the steel against (any part of) your body. In the field of nail bending, most people who have studied oldtime strongman feats would consider this technique cheating. For them, the real challenge in nail bending lies exclusively in "un-braced" bending techniques.

However, I mention it here for a very important reason: If you ever plan to perform oldtime strongman feats in front of an audience, and plan to include nail bending in your show, be advised that if you let someone from the audience test your nail, he will instinctively try to bend it on his thigh with a braced bending technique. If he is a reasonably and naturally strong man, like a carpenter or machinist, he will probably be able to kink the nail in this manner, even if he could never kink it with the "proper" underhand technique, for example. This will ruin your feat to a certain degree, as the audience does not care about the unwritten laws of the strength world and will not differentiate between these specialized techniques. All they will read into it is that any regular fellow from the street can easily "bend" your nail. Please keep this mind when you perform in front of an audience, and either set rules before you hand the nail to the audience (e.g. "Only your hands may touch the nail!"), or use a nail that is so hard to bend that not even a strong man from the street can kink it on his thigh. Either way, do give your audience the opportunity to test your nail. Otherwise, how should they know that the feat is difficult at all?

Training for any nail bending technique is easy and obvious, and one should really not make a science out of it. Three elements are essential: You should a) make sure that you regularly train all of the basic movement pattern I described in the beginning of this book, to make sure you have a great amount of general upper-body strength (especially chest strength). You should b) regularly do levering exercises for the kind of wrist strength you need, for example with a sledgehammer. Finally, and most importantly, you should c) train actual nail bending. All you have to do here is to ensure you have progression. Start out with nails that are easy to bend and gradually move up to the tougher nails. Also, you should have variation by experimenting with your technique, grip, pads, etc., until you find the parameters that work best for you.

When I started out with nail bending training for my shows, I already had a considerable amount of general strength, and did not worry about additional training for my chest, for example. All I did was go to the hardware store and buy a handful of different nails, or spikes. Luckily, the hardware store had only one *type* of nail in different lengths, which became thicker with increasing length. Thus, I did not have to do a scientific analysis of material, thickness, leverage, size standards, etc. All I had to do was to find the one size of nail that was tough enough to bend to be suitable for a show (by suitable I mean so tough that nobody in an audience could replicate the feat). I also got hold of a sledgehammer to do some levering exercises, although I did these rather half-heartedly. My focus was the actual nail bending. This I did with an underhand technique and two thick pieces of leather as pads, and with a size of nail that I could soon bend with some effort. So all I did was bend these nails, experiment with pads and technique, and, from time to time, try the next size of nail.

As the date of my first live performance kept moving closer, I did not have too much time – only a couple of weeks altogether. Eventually, I managed to bend nails one size larger then the ones I had started out with, and I was satisfied for the moment. I successfully included bending such a nail into my show. It worked well and was popular with the audience. However, I should not say that up to this point I had really *trained* for nail bending. I had only *learned* the basic technique, worked a bit on it, *tested* my nail bending strength, and determined my present maximum "weight".

Here it gets interesting, because from this moment on, my nail bending training was practically non-existent. Or, rather, my shows were my training. As I was happy with the nail I could already bend (not having much of a comparison), I focused on other things in my regular workouts. I only bent nails regularly in my shows, one at a time, every few weeks or months (I did not have many shows at that time), and then a maximum of three to four nails per day, depending on the number of shows I did per day.

Then, by and by, as the number of shows I played increased, it would occasionally happen that some sturdy fellow from the audience managed to kink the nail I had planned to bend. I realized that this was a problem. Even if the kink was minimal, it diminished the intended effect of a "superhuman" feat. Thus, I decided to go back to nail bending training. I purchased a handful of the next size of nails at the hardware store, took them with me to my home gym, warmed up, wrapped the first nail, and – *voilà* – bent it!

What had happened? It appears that I had made considerable progress and moved up to the next level of nail without any specific, targeted training: no weekly nail bending session, no sets, no repetitions, only bending my "maximum" nail every now and then. One should believe that this went against all my principles: no real progression, no real continuity, and, not to mention, any variety or partialisation. However, there is still a certain logic behind the evident progress I had made. I believe that it was owed to a phenomenon that could be called *conditioning*. By bending, with some regularity, relatively tough nails that were my "maximum" at that time (even if not every week), my body and nervous system *learned* this formerly unfamiliar movement and became *accustomed* to it.

This is a crucial aspect. Some experienced men had already observed before me that certain types of strength are *learned* rather than *built* (and are therefore easier to maintain!). It is also a commonly known fact that we humans *learn* by *repetition*. Thus, if you perform a certain movement often and regularly, even if you never increase the resistance and never go to your very limits, you will eventually become stronger in that movement. Although I do not have the evidence at hand, I am quite certain that this phenomenon is backed by science.

This is especially interesting with regard to feats of strength in which it is very hard to progress from one level to the next, because there is a large gap between these levels. It would be a worthwhile approach to such a feat of strength to simply perform it on a level you can manage well, for a long period of time, with some regularity and patience, until your body and nervous system are fairly accustomed to the movement. You do this without forcing any progression. Then, after a considerable amount of time (a year, perhaps) and a considerable amount of times of repeating the movement regularly, you try the next step. I can affirm that this works, even if it appears to contradict my four principles described above. However, it does conform to the principle of continuity, and the progression happens on a long-term scale.

To come back to my nail bending training. I took full advantage of this method once I had discovered it. Let us call it the method, or principle, of *conditioning*. Of course, I immediately started using this larger size of nail in my shows. And, as I had realized that I could become stronger in nail bending without any regular training, but simply by doing my shows, I continued in the same manner. This larger nail was now of a size and toughness that nobody from the street could bend with an un-braced bending technique (the only person I ever gave it to who managed to kink it with an underhand technique, was a strong Styrian fellow who is certified for both the Ironmind Red Nail and the Ironmind #3 hand gripper).

For the fun of it, I made the feat even harder, step by step, by reducing the pads and increasing the speed of the bend. Thus, I evidently became stronger and stronger – still without any regular training! After a few years I could fully bend this nail with absolutely minimal wrapping – a piece of leather about a millimetre thick – and without any apparent effort, but with a smile on my face. This image, combined with that of a strong volunteer from the audience, who would test the nail first and try hard, but never manage to bend it even a millimetre, always created a nice, even comical effect in front of an audience. It obviously made me appear incredibly strong, or in possession of magical powers (or a cheater!).

The nice thing about nail bending with the underhand technique is that it requires this special kind of wrist strength that takes time to build, and that most strong men do not train for. Therefore, it is one of the feats a person with a slender frame can master if he trains for it, whereas a huge bodybuilder who has never trained for it will almost certainly fail. This creates a wonderful effect for the performing oldtime strongman (although it is not very nice to shatter a bodybuilder's ego in this way). As a final note, I might add that I have once also bent the same nail without any pads at all. However, I cut my skin in doing so, which is not appropriate in front of an audience. You should not tolerate that children in the audience have to see blood. Therefore, I recommend you always use pads when bending nails in front of an audience.

As you might know, I am also certified for bending the Ironmind Red Nail. I had decided to try this at one point, to document my strength with an internationally recognized standard – even though a commercial company set this standard. I purchased a couple of Red Nails and the corresponding pads of artificial material from this company, and tried to bend the first nail with an underhand technique. However, I failed. Thus, I concluded that bending this piece of steel with an underhand technique is quite a challenge, and decided to try the technique that most successful Red Nail benders use, which is the overhand technique.

As I had never tried this technique before, and as I wanted to achieve this feat quickly to get it over with, I decided to start regular nail bending training again, rather than relying on the *conditioning* that had happened automatically with my underhand technique. I did levering exercises with a sledgehammer, this time focusing on the wrist strength needed to lever a sledgehammer *upwards* when holding it in front of you. Wanting not to make things too complicated, all I did were three or four sets of levering the sledgehammer for as many repetitions as I could, while holding it at the farthest end of the handle. For my specialized nail bending training I had purchased a few of the smaller nails of that company, including the so-called Blue Nails. For some time I did nothing else but bend a few of these nails in my training once a week, while experimenting with the pads, or wraps, and my technique.

Unfortunately, it took me some time to realize that the correct technique was the *pushing* motion I described above, rather than a *bending* motion, which I had used in my training so far. If I had realized this earlier, I would probably have saved a lot of time. Nevertheless, I believe that through all the bending I did with this "wrong", or rather *less efficient* technique, I had built a fair amount of the necessary wrist strength. Once I had discovered the proper technique, I realized how easy short steel bending in the overhand manner actually is. Believe it or not, after this discovery (and after months of training with the wrong technique), I eventually bent a Red Nail the first time I tried! Albeit, this bend was still above the time limit of one minute, and with rubber bands fixing the pads, which is not allowed in an official certification.

So I still had some way to go. By then, I had luckily realized that I would not have to purchase the Blue Nails again and again, in particular as these are too different from the Red Nail to make for a very efficient training. Instead, I would simply take regular nails from my hardware store, with a similar *thickness* as the Red Nail, and cut off the ends (the point and the head), so that they would have a similar *length* as the Red Nail. These were perfect, as they were a bit easier to bend than an actual Red Nail – probably owed to a different type of steel – but still much harder than a Blue Nail. After a few weeks of training with these, I was ready for certification.

In sum, bending nails is a solid feat of strength and an interesting endeavour that seems to turn some of the laws of strength training upside down. If one was to start nail bending training today, I would recommend the following procedure: One day per week for nail bending training, consisting of two exercises: sledgehammer levering for general wrist strength and as a warm-up, and actual nail bending training with nails you can bend tolerably well. With these nails, you do a number of "single repetitions" (meaning bending one nail once), while you constantly experiment with the technique, grip, and pads, to find out what works best for you. You do this continuously for weeks and months. Every once in a while, you try to move up a step by trying a bigger nail, or try a different possibility for progression in smaller steps: you use the same nails and cut a little bit off at one end to make them shorter, which makes the feat more difficult as it reduces the leverage. This is basically all. The biggest deciding factors in your nail bending training will be, by every means, time and technique. It is entirely up to you if you want to train several bending styles at the same time, go for only one style at a time, or even decide which style is best for you and then stick with this style only.

One more thing I should probably mention here, although I want to discuss it in more detail later, is the mental aspect in nail bending. Nail bending is an integral part of my show, and I have never failed to bend a nail I wanted to bend in any of my shows. However, it has happened several times in my *training* that when I wanted to bend a nail I had regularly bent before, just to test if I still had the strength (for example at the beginning of a new show season), I could not! However, once I stepped on a *stage* after this, I could bend the same nail as easily as butter – although it was the same *me*, the same *body*, that is to say, the same *physical matter*, that tried to bend the nail. Also, mind you that I usually never *train* for nail bending now, but when I try to bend one in front of an audience, I never *fail*. I have bent such nails before audiences in the pouring rain, in the gleaming sun, and in icy winters, always bare-chested (because I always perform bare-chested). Sometimes I have done shows without even warming up and bent nails in them (which is not a very wise thing to do). Still, in training, even under the best conditions, I have occasionally failed.

From this, I conclude that there is a large mental aspect in nail bending (as in most feats of strength, for that matter). Whenever I *have* to bend a nail that I *know* I can bend in theory, I succeed. And in front of an audience, you *have* to, because otherwise your show is ruined. Now, if you could develop a similar attitude in training, or at least for your record attempts, I believe it could help you a lot. Again, there are two aspects to this attitude: *having* to succeed, and *knowing* that the nail can be bent, or rather that *you* can bend it.

However, I am not saying that it is easy to develop this kind of attitude in training. In a training situation it is fake and artificial: You do not actually *have* to bend the nail, because nothing will happen if you fail. The world will just keep turning. Therefore, if you successfully develop this attitude in training, you are cheating on yourself, in a way.

Knowing that the nail can be bent is interesting, because when you witness someone trying to bend a big nail for the first time, you realize that, after their first go, their mind tells them that this feat is impossible, and their strength is gone – even if they give it a second go. They do not utilize their full potential, because they lack the *knowledge* that it is humanly possible – they simply do not believe in it (any more). However, as I *know* that the steel can be bent, because I have bent it hundreds of times before, my mind allows me to utilize its full potential.

This is crucial in nail bending, by the way: The ability to exert full force in one moment. Bending the toughest nail you can theoretically bend, requires a surge of energy that is singular. Everything has to come together. There is no rising curve, no initial phase. Once the bend begins, all your potential force has to be exerted at one go. Being able to channel your strength and energy in this way, is a skill that requires practice, experience, and concentration. Therefore, I believe in remaining calm and concentrated before a feat of strength. In my opinion, loud screaming, display behaviour, and the like, already expend some of your energy. Such behaviour is energy that *leaves* your body, and you should aim at the opposite: to *conserve* as much energy as possible inside your body, channel it, and release into the feat of strength at one singular moment. I am sorry if this sounds transcendental or esoteric, but if you try this for a long enough period of time, maybe you will realize what I am talking about. Do not be discouraged if you fail the first couple of times, as this skill does not come easily, but over time.

9.4. Horseshoe bending

The bending of horseshoes is really one of my favourite oldtime strongman feats. A horseshoe is an interesting object, the bending technique is cunning, and the feat has something very nostalgic and archaic about it – reminding us of the times when horses were part of our everyday lives. Much of what I said about nail bending can also be said about horseshoe bending. Both are steel bending feats, both require the singular extortion of full force, it is difficult to have progression in both, and both require grip and wrist strength. Some of the differences between horseshoe bending and nail bending are that horseshoes are much more interesting objects than nails, that horseshoe bending is a visually more pleasing feat, that horseshoes are more expensive and harder to get, that it is more of an asymmetrical load for the body, and that horseshoe bending is almost always a feat that belongs to the category of "braced bending", meaning you stabilize the horseshoe against your hip in the initial phase, and push it against your thigh in the final phase (or, if you want to bend it the full 360 degrees, the "final" phase consists of squeezing it between your thighs).

In horseshoe bending, much depends on the technique, which is a little bit more complex than in nail bending. It is actually the unfamiliarity with the technique that makes most people fail the first time they try to bend a horseshoe. This being said, even when one has mastered the technique, a tough horseshoe remains a tremendous challenge. This is also why the feat is so famous, because it is *really* difficult to do if the horseshoe has a tolerable thickness and strength of material.

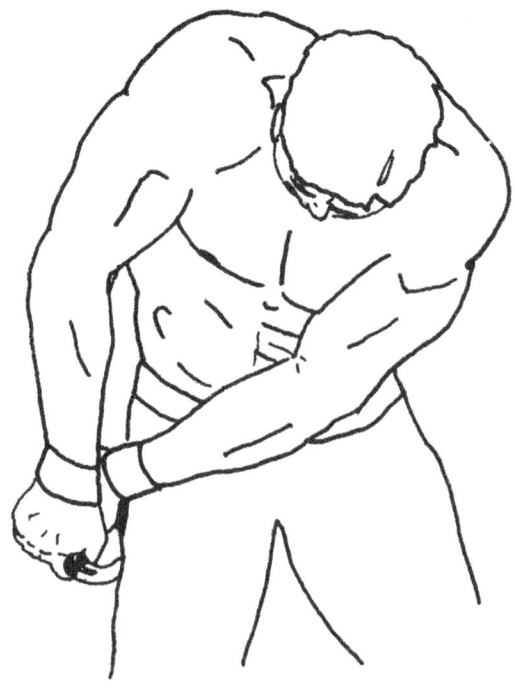

Figure 9.10 Horseshoe bending.

84

Let me start by talking a little bit about the technique of this feat – although no words can explain it as well as seeing the feat in actual life, or in a film, or someone demonstrating and explaining it to you in person. In his book *Feats of Strength and Dexterity*, Charles McMahon explains the technique in the following manner:

> "[G]rasp the two ends, one in each hand, and holding it on your thigh push with one hand or arm and pull with the other. If nothing happens, try twisting it in half by pushing one end down and the other up instead of directly away from each other as in the previous method." (McMahon 92)

Although this is correct in principle, the description can be somewhat misleading. First of all, it is important to make clear which hand is placed where. Let us assume you are right-handed. Then your left hand would hold onto the one end of the horseshoe close to your hip, in a manner that the "centre" of the horseshoe rests against your thigh, or, rather, *behind* your thigh. Thus, your left arm reaches across your whole torso and holds the horseshoe in place on your right hip. Left hand and arm are not supposed to move during the initial phase of the bend, but are rather only meant to keep the horseshoe where it is. It comes near to a pulling movement, albeit without any real motion. The right hand then grabs the other end of the horseshoe. This hand is supposed to move, as it must push down on the other end of the horseshoe, i.e. push it down and back, towards your right heel, away from the body. This is what Mr McMahon means by "twisting it in half by pushing one end down and the other up" in his second method. You have to cause a torsion in the horseshoe with an "S"-shape as the result. An illustration of a bent horseshoe will explain better what I mean than any words:

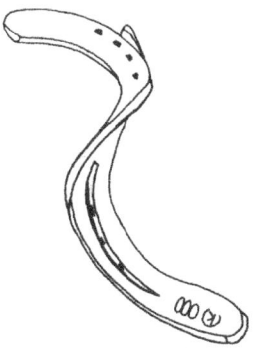

Figure 9.11 A horseshoe bent to 180 degrees.

As a consequence, much of the feat depends on grip strength. It can become quite a challenge to hold the horseshoe tightly enough to keep from twisting in your hands. This would make the desired torsion impossible.

Holding the horseshoe with one hand and pushing down with the other is not the whole story, though. A tough horseshoe requires a great amount of strength from the core. While you push down on the farther end, your torso and lower body should move closer, you should almost double up. A major part of the force required to push down on the farther end should come from this movement rather than just from your right arm. Both your arms will remain bent during this phase, also your right arm, although it will eventually almost straighten.

Once you have mastered the initial bend – let us say once you have bent, or opened up, the horseshoe to about 90 degrees – a second phase follows. In this phase, you place the centre of the horseshoe on your (in this case right) thigh, near to the hip, and push down on the ends with both hands. While doing this, you should flex your quadriceps muscle. Once the horseshoe is bent, or opened, to nearly 180 degrees, it can be considered fully bent. However, some would say it has to be bent at least slightly past 180 degrees to be considered a good bend.

Although I would argue that the initial bend is always the hardest part in horseshoe bending, and the following second phase, where you push down on the ends, is relatively easy, compared to it, I should add that depending of the shoe, the very end of the second phase can become exceedingly difficult again, especially as you are nearing the 180 degrees, or try to go beyond them.

Following the second phase, there is an optional third phase. In the third phase you push even farther down on the ends of the horseshoe until it is bent *way beyond* 180 degrees. Then you put the horseshoe between your thighs, where you push the ends farther together with chest strength through the hands, and with adductor strength through the thighs. Once the shoe is, technically, bent to about "360 degrees", the bend is complete.

Personally, I am not so fond of bending horseshoes beyond 180 degrees, because this is only possible with lighter horseshoes that do not require your full potential for the initial bent. Therefore, I prefer tougher horseshoes that I can only bend to a maximum of 180 degrees (or just slightly beyond that).

However, there is a good reason for bending horseshoes to 360 degrees if you want to perform in front of an audience. Once bent to 360 degrees, the horseshoe naturally acquires a curious shape that is reminiscent of a heart. It therefore becomes a nice item you can hand to a woman in the audience as a keepsake, or to a man, depending on your preference. To avoid confusions you could also say it is meant to be a pretzel.

If we analyse the proper horseshoe bending technique, we realise that this feat requires strength from a great variety of body parts and muscle groups: grip strength and wrist strength, pulling strength in the left arm (i.e. biceps and latissimus), pushing strength in the right arm for the initial phase and in both arms for the second phase (i.e. triceps and chest), a strong core (i.e. abdominal muscles) and, if you care to go beyond 180 degrees, strength in the legs, i.e. in the adductors. In sum, one could say it is a true full-body exercise. In addition to this, you require a degree of pain tolerance: in your hands, as well as in your thigh for the second, pushing-down phase.

It should go without saying that pads, or wraps, are also needed for the tougher horseshoes you want to bend. Especially when you start out with horseshoe bending training you should always use pads. Later on, when you have mastered a specific, light horseshoe, you can gradually reduce the pads and eventually leave them away to make the feat even harder. But again: When you start out, wrap the ends of the horseshoe in leather and put a piece of leather on your thigh, at least for the push-down phase, but perhaps also for the initial bend. I am saying leather, because I prefer to use natural materials wherever possible. Of course, there are many who prefer an artificial material they have found works particularly well for them instead.

Here, the same rule as for nail bending applies: You will have to experiment with different materials, degrees of thickness, and so on, until you find out what works best for you. I prefer a relatively thin but stiff type of leather for the ends of the horseshoe, and a thick and even sturdier type of leather for the thigh. Soft leather, which is highly flexible, is not very useful. Also, wrap the ends of the horseshoe as tightly as possible (the same is true for nail bending). It might help if you scatter some chalk onto the leather and the shoe before you wrap it, and to keep the wraps in place with rubber bands, to keep them from loosening (you can remove these rubber bands right before the bend if you wish).

If your wraps are so large that they stick out a little bit beyond the ends of the horseshoe, this increases your leverage to a certain degree. It is not considered cheating if it is not overdone. However, thicker pads are not necessarily better. The pads should neither be too thick nor too long, so as not to increase the diameter of your "handles" too much when wrapped around them. This would create a kind of crush zone that absorbs some of the force you try to exert on your bend. Talking about the exertion of force, what I said about the mental aspect in nail bending above, applies to horseshoes equally well.

A big question mark in horseshoe bending is where to get the horseshoes from. Here you have two possibilities: used or new horseshoes. I would recommend you start with used horseshoes, because they are practically available in unlimited quantities, for free, and in a great variety of shapes and sizes. This will allow you to learn and experiment with your technique. Also, some used horseshoes, if well-worn, will be very easy to bend. This will inspire a sense of achievement early on in your training and demystify the feat of bending a horseshoe.

However, to get hold of used horseshoes, you will have to go out into the real world and talk to people. You will have to go to a riding stable, a farrier, or the like, and ask the people there if they can spare a couple of used horseshoes. Usually they will give them away gladly because used horseshoes accrue regularly, and are of no use to these people any more. Of course, they will ask you what you need them for, and if you are embarrassed about your horseshoe bending plans and oldtime strongman training, you could say that you need them for decoration, or that you are an artist and need them for a piece of art. In sum, I suggest this approach when you start out, because it is cost neutral and because worn horseshoes are in principle easier to bend.

This being said, there are also some types of new horseshoes that are easier to bend then some used ones. If you find out which, you can find the next horseshoe supplier and ask them for these particular types. Or, preferably, you personally visit your next horseshoe supplier and ask them for guidance. Obviously, they do not produce and distribute horseshoes for the purpose of being bent, and will have no experience with regard to which types are easy or hard to bend. But they will be able to tell you something about the different types of steel and the different sizes available. Apart from the type of steel, which only an expert can determine, there are a few other parameters that decide whether a horseshoe is easy or hard to bend, *viz.*:

♦ Thickness: The thinner and narrower the shoe is, the easier it is to bend.

♦ Size: This is somewhat counter-intuitive. A larger horseshoe is in principle easier to bend than a smaller one, because it gives you greater leverage. However, larger horseshoes are usually thicker as well, so this rule only applies if you compare two horseshoes that are equally thick, but differ in size. In such a case, the larger horseshoe will be easier to bend.

♦ Clips: Many horseshoes have so-called clips – small, half-circular protrusions, either one at the centre (usually for the front hoofs) or two at the sides (usually for the rear hoofs). Any clipped horseshoe is harder to bend than the same shoe without clips. The reasons for this are obvious: A front-clip adds material to the centre, i.e. the part where the horseshoe is supposed to give in, and side-clips add a little bit of general stability to the shoe and reduce the surface to hold onto at the ends. Also, a front-clip requires greater pain tolerance in your thigh in the second phase of the bend, because you actually push the clip into your quadriceps muscle. For these reasons I suggest you start out with un-clipped horseshoes if possible, and, if you want, progress to clipped shoes later on.

There are lists of horseshoe types from different companies and in different sizes, arranged in a rough order of "easy to bend" to "extremely difficult to bend". I do not want to copy and paste such a list here and sell it as my own idea, but with a thorough search you should be able to find it. This will be tremendously helpful for you to make a start (i.e. to find a horseshoe that is easy to bend to begin with) and to make progression (i.e. to find harder and harder horseshoes as you move up the ladder).

However, mind you that such a list is never absolute. Companies that produce horseshoes might change materials, take certain horseshoes out of their product range, or go bankrupt altogether. I, for example, started out with horseshoes from the Dutch company Werkman, but eventually my horseshoe supplier stopped distributing these, or the company stopped producing them – I am not sure. I then switched to horseshoes from the Dutch company Kerckhaert and have used these ever since.

I am not particularly fond of trying too many different horseshoes from too many different companies, as I always try to keep things simple. In actual fact, I have only used Kerckheart horseshoes of the type "sx 7". These are relatively well known among horseshoe benders in our present times. A specific size of this type of horseshoe, the size "000" with side-clips, is an acknowledged benchmark. In actual fact, this is the hardest horseshoe I have bent so far as I am writing this: a Kerckheart sx 7, size 000, with side-clips. These sx 7 shoes also have the advantage that they are available in a very clear order of progression in terms of size, indicated by the number after the "sx 7". This number is clearly printed on one end of the shoe. The smallest size is the triple zero – "000" – and therefore the hardest to bend. A size "1", for example, is comparatively easy to bend, but still a challenge. For a beginner, it can appear as a feat impossible to achieve. Size "1" is followed by "0", "00", and, finally "000". Any of these sizes is available with or without clips, but with clips it is harder to bend.

All of this does not mean that you have to use horseshoes from the same company or of the same type. All I am trying to say is that it helps if you find a type of horseshoe that is continuously available and allows progression in your training. Ideally, it is also well known among horseshoe benders, so that you can measure your progress against that of others.

However, this is not a must if you want to train for this feat to perform it live. In this case, you only have to find a horseshoe that is so hard to bend that a regular person from the street cannot do anything with it.

Even if you do find a type of horseshoe that is available in different sizes and allows you to progress from one to the next in clear steps, these steps might be considerable. For example, if you can bend a "Kerckheart sx 7, size 0" horseshoe this week, a size "00" can still appear impossible the week after. Above, in the chapter "How to get better at any feat of strength", I already mentioned some of the methods to ensure progression in horseshoe bending in smaller steps. To quickly mention them again here, one possibility is to cut a certain amount of millimetres into the centre of a horseshoe with a hacksaw, making it slightly easier to bend. Then you reduce the number of millimetres step by step. However, this is not a very exact method. A different possibility would be to use iron pipes you can put onto the ends of a horseshoe, to make the "handles" slightly longer and increase the leverage. In this way you will be able to bend horseshoes you cannot bend regularly. It has the advantage that it will demystify these horseshoes, but it has the disadvantage that you will not be able to practice the proper grip. In any way, your creativity is called upon to find a way to progress with horseshoes.

You can also apply the principle of partialisation to horseshoe bending training. For example, you can pry open a certain horseshoe with a vice, to skip the first phase of the bend and start out with the second phase. I would recommend you do this right after you have pried it open in the vice, because the metal will heat up during the bend, making it easier to bend it further. Once it has cooled down after the first phase of the bend, the second phase will be even harder.

As with nail bending, it is impossible to train horseshoe bending with sets of repetitions, as any horseshoe bend is one set of one repetition. Therefore, you might be able to make progress with the phenomenon of conditioning. If you simply bend enough horseshoes over time – even if you always use the same type of shoe – your body and nervous system will eventually adapt to the involved movements and internalise them. Gradually, over time, your standard horseshoe will become easier to bend. One day you will be able to take a great step and progress to the next horseshoe in line, which is considerably harder to bend. This method requires the principle of continuity, and, thus, patience. Whichever method you decide to use, it is crucial that you work systematically.

9.5. Grip strength feats

Grip strength training is a huge chapter in oldtime strongman training. One could probably build an entire strongman career based on grip strength feats alone. There are not only countless variations on grip strength feats. Grip strength is also considered a primary indicator of general body strength. And reversely, overall body strength seems to benefit from a strong grip. This might be the reason why a strong grip and grip strength feats have always been considered indicators of general strength and great physical ability in many cultural contexts. Furthermore, our hands and their abilities are also inherently human, as hardly any kind of animal has the dexterity and versatility in its hands that we humans have. Next to us humans, only primates have similarly versatile hands, but they do not use them with the great sophistication as we humans do (this being said, apes like chimpanzees and gorillas have much *stronger* hands than we humans – we have to give them credit for this).

As mentioned above, I have written a whole book about grip strength training, together with the strongman Tommy Heslep (at the moment I am writing this, Mr Heslep is one in only five persons in the whole world who successfully certified for the Ironmind #4 hand gripper). Thus, as grip strength training already filled this whole book (and other books as well), I do not want to go into too much detail here and limit myself to a few crucial aspects.

Because our hands are so versatile, their possibilities for movement and the ways to train them, and demonstrate their ability in feats of strength, are manifold. I talk a little bit about this in my book *Grip Strength,* but from a very general and systematic training approach (although I also mention in this book how to train for some common feats of grip strength). To complement the information provided in *Grip Strength*, I want to take a slightly different approach here and talk, first and foremost, about hand strength for show purposes.

I believe that the myriad of grip strength feats can be categorized into four different types of feats, which I will explain below:

1. Lifting feats
2. Obstacle handle feats
3. Dynamic grip strength feats
4. Secondary grip strength feats

Ad 1): By *lifting feats* I mean any kind of lifting strength feat where hand strength is the limiting factor – whether the feat is advertised as such (e.g. a one-finger lift, the asset of which is obviously the great strength of a single finger, making it an obvious feat of grip strength even to an uninformed audience) or not (e.g. lifting the Dinnie Stones – a feat that, to a layman, appears difficult because of the great weight of the stones, while many do not know that hand strength is the weak link in this feat). What all lifting feats have in common, however, is that it is not considered cheating if the handle to hold onto has an ideal shape to exert full finger strength. For example, if you do a one-finger lift, you may use the kind of handle that allows you the best possible grip. Depending on your preference, what I define as "handle" can be anything like a metal ring of varying thickness, a leather band, a piece of rope, or whatever. The reason for this being that nobody will ask whether the handle you used was comfortable or not, or a disadvantage or not. People will only ask whether you managed the one-finger lift or not. The asset in lifting feats will be the number of kilograms (or pounds) lifted, either with one, two, three, etc. fingers, or with one whole hand (once you use two hands, though, the limiting factor will probably not be hand strength any more).

As a consequence, the feats I categorize as lifting feats mostly have in common that the hand, or the individual fingers, will tend to be rather closed. A closed hand, holding onto a relatively "thin" handle, can exert more strength than an open hand, holding onto a thick handle. This being said, there is probably an ideal (individual) thickness for any handle that will feel most comfortable for you and allow you to mobilize your maximum hand strength (a handle that is too thin will hurt and make the feat more difficult again).

To sum up, classic lifting feats are one-hand lifts and one-finger lifts. A two-finger lift might be performed to some effect, whereas a three-finger lift is already rather pointless. Also one-arm pull-ups, all the way up to one-finger pull-ups, should be categorized as lifting feats according to this definition. These also confirm the rule that it is not so much the shape of the pull-up bar that defines this feat, but the fact in itself that someone is able to pull ("lift") his bodyweight up with one hand (or one finger, etc.).

Ad 2): *Obstacle handle feats* are related to lifting feats in so far as they are also *lifts* most of the time. However, the difference is that the defining aspect of obstacle handle feats is the handle that is particularly hard to hold onto, e.g. a thick handled dumbbell. This makes their asset not so much the sheer poundage of the weight lifted, but rather the fact that someone is able to lift the specified weight at all – given such an uncomfortable handle. An obstacle handle feat can be impressive, even if the lifted weight is rather low – as long as the handle makes this low amount of weight exceedingly difficult to lift. A perfect example would be the historic feat of the Austrian Franz Föttinger, who, in 1896, lifted a weight of 12kg (26lbs), only by a sewing needle that he would squeeze between his thumb and index finger. The needle was hammered into a piece of wood to which the weight was attached. Although the weight was not particularly heavy, nobody could replicate his feat.

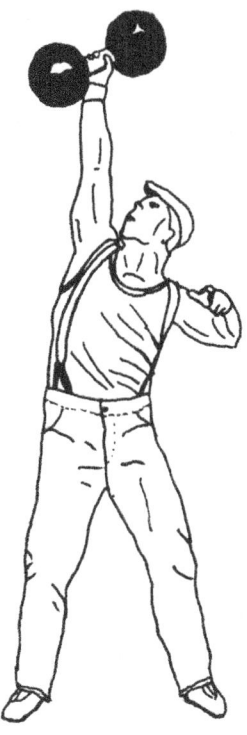

Figure 9.12 An Inch-style dumbbell lifted overhead.

This very specialized feat is of course an exception. The most popular and well-known obstacle handle feats involve thick handles, i.e. handles that require a rather open hand. The most famous historical feat of this kind is the dumbbell of the British oldtime strongman Thomas Inch, which is known as "Inch dumbbell" in our days. It weighed 78kg (172lbs). Replicas and similar models in different weight categories are available nowadays. Such a dumbbell can be simply deadlifted, or cleaned, and/or (push-) pressed. Although it might not be obvious to a layman in an audience, the limiting factor in this feat is the hand strength. Anyone who will try to lift such a thick handled dumbbell off the floor with one hand for the first time (and fail), and then with two hands, simply to check the weight (and succeed), will realize this soon. Even the original Inch dumbbell would be relatively easy to lift with one hand if the handle was thinner, as the weight itself is not incredibly heavy.

Similar things could be said of any type of "Apollon's Axle" lift. This is a barbell with a very thick bar, very difficult to lift, although it is meant to be lifted with two hands (usually with a parallel grip).

Also the wide variety of pinch grip feats belong into the category of obstacle handle feats, as they usually involve a challenge to pinch grip an object and lift it, with the weight being not particularly heavy in itself, but the lifting very hard to do because of the way one holds onto it. This being said, the needle lift of Franz Föttinger is also a pinch grip lift.

Ad 3): *Dynamic grip strength feats* I define as feats that involve an object manipulation through the closing of the hand. In other words, these feats might be called "crushing feats", as they usually involve an object being crushed. The best and most vivid example is crushing an everyday object like an apple (easy) or a potato (difficult). Other than in lifting and obstacle handle feats, the grip is not static. Such feats can emphasize the whole hand, to exert maximum force, or the thumbs, for example when trying to crush a walnut with the thumb.

Ad 4): What I mean by *secondary grip strength feats* are such that involve a large amount of grip strength, but also strength from other muscle groups to a large extent, so that they cannot be considered purely *grip strength feats*. Examples would be steel bending feats, like nail bending, which require great grip strength, but wrist strength as well. But also feats like card tearing or phone book tearing are principally grip strength feats, but involve other types of strength as well, which is why I would like to put them in this same category.

Here is a categorization of some popular and well-known feats of grip strength according to my system:

1. Lifting feats:
   ◆ One-finger lift, two-finger lift, etc.
   ◆ One-hand lift
   ◆ Dinnie Stones
   ◆ One-hand pull-up
   ◆ One-finger pull-up, two-finger pull-up, etc.

2. Obstacle handle feats:
- Inch dumbbell lift
- "Apollon's Axle" lift
- Lifting barbell plates with a pinch grip (e.g. two 20kg (44lbs) plates)
- Lifting barbell plate by the hub
- Lifting anvil by the horn
- "Needle lift"

3. Dynamic grip strength feats:
- Crushing an apple in one hand
- Crushing a raw potato in one hand
- Crushing walnuts
- Crushing cans of beer
- Bending beer bottle top with fingers

4. Secondary grip strength feats:
- Tearing decks of cards
- Tearing phone books
- Nail bending
- Horseshoe bending
- Sledgehammer levering

This is quite a number of feats, but still only a selection. There are also some grip strength feats that cannot be clearly categorized according to my scheme. In any case, if one has a strong grip, he is qualified for a wide range of classic and modern strongman feats. In fact, a whole, varied strongman performance could be designed out of a choice of these feats.

Albeit, you should not think that training for one grip strength feat qualifies you to do all of them. The different categories of grip strength feats require different methods of training. Nobody will doubt that someone who can lift 150kg (331lbs) with one finger has a strong grip, but this does not mean that he will be able to deadlift an Inch dumbbell replica as well. There are some correlations, however. Someone who can lift an Inch dumbbell replica, will also do well on an Apollon's Axle, and will probably also have a strong pinch grip. The reason for this is that most *obstacle handle feats* require great strength from the *thumb* and *fingertips*, which is not the primary requirement of a feat that is performed with a *closed hand*. Vice versa, if someone is good at *lifting feats* with one (closed) hand, he will also be good at lifting with the strongest finger of this hand (the middle finger). But neither of these require a movement of the hand across a range of motion, like the *dynamic grip strength* feats.

Below, in the chapter "Setting priorities", I will talk about focalization in training. If you follow my advice, you will approach feats of grip strength in groups according to my categorization. That is, if you really want to make progress in one particular type of feat. On the other hand, if you simply want to build a generally strong grip, not with any *particular* feat in mind, you should include exercises in your training regimen that cover at least all of the first three categories. In the following, I will explain some possibilities of how to train for these.

Ad 1): *Lifting feats* require a strong, static grip with a closed hand. The advantage of this kind of strength is that it can be trained automatically, while you train other muscle groups or movement patterns. The best example is the regular deadlift. It is always a good idea for any aspiring old-time strongman to make the deadlift a fixed part of one's regimen.

However, not many people know that performing heavy deadlifts each week, close to one's maximum, is counterproductive. Heavy deadlifts are a great stress for your whole locomotor and nervous system and are best trained by the principle of partialisation, or by the principle of conditioning I explained above. You can kill two birds with one stone when you apply the latter: You can perform regular deadlifts with a moderate weight, while seriously training your grip, if you perform deadlifts with *grip variations*. For example: if you do deadlifts with a double overhand grip, you will not be able to lift as much as you could with a mixed grip. But you will train your grip (which will be the weak link in this exercise if you use a parallel overhand grip) and *condition* your body for the deadlift movement at the same time. The week after, you could do the same with a four-finger deadlift (only index fingers and middle fingers of each hand), either with a parallel overhand, or a reverse grip. The week after, you do deadlifts only with your middle fingers, and so on. You can also try one-hand deadlifts on a regular barbell. Then, every once in a while, you can switch to a reverse grip with both hands (the kind of grip that allows you to lift your maximum deadlift weight) to measure your progress in the deadlift. This is probably the best method to make progress in the deadlift and in lifting grip strength at the same time. In this manner, both will benefit from each other. Hermann Görner, perhaps the best natural deadlifter in history, used a similar method.

I should also add here that I recommend you do all your deadlifting training with a barbell with only minimal knurling (except, perhaps, for your maximum attempts). The reason for this is twofold: a) Less knurling will require more grip strength and train your hand more effectively. b) A bar with coarse knurling, although allowing you to lift greater weights, is more prone to rip open the skin of your hands. This you obviously want to avoid, as you might have to pause with your training on certain feats until the skin has healed.

Not all are aware that a regular barbell, although it is designed to have a thickness that is comfortable for most to hold in their hands, does not allow you to lift your maximum weight one-handed (or with one finger, for that matter). One reason for this is that an Olympic barbell has a revolving handle, and a non-revolving handle would be much easier to hold onto. The more important reason, however, is that for a maximum one-hand lift you would require a narrower handle. This is because most human hands can exert greater strength in a lifting motion if the hand is slightly more closed than a regular barbell allows.

The ring on the Dinnie Stones, for example, is much more suitable for a one-hand lift than a regular barbell. If you wanted to train for your maximum one-hand lift, you should find some kind of handle that feels comfortable to you. In all likelihood, this will consist of a metal bar (or ring), slightly narrower than a regular barbell (but mind you that you will have to think creatively of a way to fix weight to this ring, as a regularly strong man will soon be able to lift a considerable amount of weight in this manner – exceeding 100kg (221lbs) by far).

The same is true for a one- or two-finger lift. A one-finger lift on a regular barbell is exceedingly difficult, and much easier with a sling of rope, for example. I am not saying that this makes a one-hand or one-finger lift less painful. In fact, pain tolerance plays a large role in these kinds of feats. If holding on to your narrow handle in training is painful, mind you that becoming used to this pain is part of the training for such feats.

There is another wonderful possibility to train for the kind of strength and pain tolerance one-hand and one-finger lifts require, while you train another movement pattern at the same time. These are pull-ups on a narrow bar, or on slings of rope. On such, you can do regular pull-ups, pull-ups with three, two, or one finger(s) per hand, or, if you are able to, one-hand pull-ups. All of these will build your hand strength and pain tolerance for lifting feats, while training your "climbing" muscles (latissimus, biceps, trapezius...) at the same time.

One more note here: to lift the highest possible weight with one hand, even on a narrow handle, one should use a hook grip. In a hook grip, the thumb lies beneath the fingers of the hand, and is squeezed in such a manner that there is a mechanical barrier to the opening of your hand, and not just a barrier depending on your muscle strength (Olympic weightlifters regularly use this grip). Some might consider this cheating, but most will not. It requires even greater pain tolerance.

Ad 2): As explained above, the idea behind *obstacle handle feats* is not to lift a maximum weight, but to lift a smaller weight, albeit with a more difficult grip. As a principle, one could say all obstacle handle feats represent a considerable "deviation from the norm", i.e. from the type of grip that allows you to lift the maximum weight possible. As the human hand can lift the most weight with a rather closed hand, as explained above, it follows that most obstacle handles require rather opened hands, and thus more strength from the fingertips and thumb. This is also true of the "needle lift", although this feat is an exception that represents the opposite end of the spectrum of obstacle handle feats, with a hand closed to the utmost.

If you want to train for obstacle handle feats, it would be wise to find a way to effectively train fingertips and thumbs. This can be done with very specific training, with some feat of strength in mind, for example deadlifts with a thick barbell. This is no a bad choice, because it is straightforward and simple and allows easy progression. All you have to do is add weight plates to the bar. Such a bar can be purchased from a specialised dealer, or one can simply use a metal pipe with a thick diameter (50mm (2in) would be the first choice, as this is also the diameter of Olympic barbell plates and will allow you to load corresponding weights) and clamps on both sides to resemble a regular barbell. A regular pipe of this kind should be sturdy enough to hold the maximum weight a strong man can lift with such a thick handled bar. A further advantage of this training is that it can be utilised as conditioning for your regular deadlift training, just as the grip variations described above in the section on lifting feats.

Similarly as with lifting strength, you can train for obstacle handle feats with pull-ups, if you use a thick bar. I believe that a fixed thick bar for pull-ups is of limited use, though, as it will only require little more grip strength than a regular pull-up bar. You will thus soon reach a level where your grip strength is no longer the limiting factor in this exercise, but, as with regular pull-ups, your back and biceps strength. However, the exercise becomes slightly more effective for training your grip strength if you use a *revolving* thick bar. This can easily be done if you take the same tick bar or metal pipe you might use for deadlifts (see above) and let it rest on two parallel bars in a power rack, for example. Then, if you hold onto the bar for pull-ups, it will tend to roll out of your hand, making it much more difficult for you to hold onto, and thus train your grip more effectively.

Of course, such a thick bar can be used for all kinds of exercises. There are actually proponents of using a thick handle for any regular exercise, in the belief that you will automatically strengthen your grip while you train all sorts of movement patterns and muscle groups – for example barbell rows or biceps curls, but even the bench press, the shoulder press, and so on. However, I do not believe this method beneficial for oldtime strongman training. In German we have the saying "*Nicht Fisch und nicht Fleisch*", roughly translating to "Neither fish nor meat" in English, and meaning a bad compromise, which is inferior to both of the two choices. And this is exactly what you have when you do every exercise with a thick handle: It is neither the most effective grip training, nor is it the most effective way to train other muscle groups.

Therefore, I recommend you keep the two separate. Train your grip with a clear focus and straightforward exercises (like deadlifts with a thick bar), and do your other exercises with a regular barbell if you want to become better in them. The only exercises I would do with a thick bar are deadlifts, pull-ups, and, perhaps, wrist curls, reverse wrist curls, and reverse biceps curls. Regular biceps curls, barbell rows, and all other exercises are best trained with a regular barbell.

You can, of course, also include exercises in your regimen that train your *fingertips* more directly. My two favourite exercises here are pull-ups on the fingertips and pinch grip lifts. The first are effective and easy to perform; all you have to find is some kind of edge that has the proper height and sturdiness to hold your bodyweight and do pull-ups on. If you are a climber, or if climbing is a popular sport in your area, you will probably not have a hard time finding a hangboard or campus board, on which you can train your fingertips and grip with a great variety of handles and from different angles. Once you have developed a considerable amount of hand strength, you can do pull-ups on three or less fingertips per hand as well.

Then, there is a myriad of ways and contraptions to train your pinch grip – objects and handles in all shapes and sizes. As I like to keep things simple, I have built myself two tools that allow me to train my pinch grip in a straightforward way. I have designed two wooden blocks of different width (one about 50mm (2in) wide, the other about 85mm (3.3in) wide) and screwed metal hooks into the bottom of each. When I attach weight to these hooks, I can train my pinch grip in two variations (wide grip and close grip) simply by doing lifts or holds for time. The simplest way to attach weight to the hook is with a sturdy bucket you fill with stones or weights. In this manner it is easy to make progress in this exercise, as you simply increase the weight step by step. I have described this method in my book *Grip Strength* as well, and it was co-author Tommy Heslep who gave me this idea.

Ad 3): The best and most obvious way to train for *dynamic grip strength feats* is with hand grippers. To make serious progress in this kind of grip strength you need a hand gripper that offers a great amount of resistance and is very tough to squeeze. Such hand grippers are now available in a sturdy quality from a number of companies. Typically, these companies offer a progressing range of grippers, going from relatively easy to so tough that only a handful of people in the world can squeeze the handles together, or no human at all (only perhaps a gorilla if you could convince one to try). This being said, when you train with such a gripper it is generally only regarded a proper repetition if you squeeze it together so that the handles touch.

The most well-known hand grippers of this kind are manufactured by the company Ironmind. Traditionally, they produced four different strengths, specified by an Arabic numeral: the #1, #2, #3 and #4 hand grippers, with the #4 being the toughest. Not too long ago, the company also introduced intermediate steps – the #0.5, #1.5, and so on – and even lighter grippers for beginners and to warm up. Still, these grippers, as those from other companies, make progression quite difficult, as moving from one gripper to the next is often quite a large step. As a very rough rule of thumb, you will be able to do about 20 full repetitions on one particular gripper before you will be able to close the next full step of gripper, or about ten repetitions before you will be able to move to the next half-step.

As the principle of progression should be applied in dynamic grip strength feats and the training of such, this can become a problem. I will talk more about this later. But I should also mention here that there are, of course, other training tools that can do a similar job as these kinds of grippers. There are grippers where the resistance can be increased and decreased in smaller steps, simply by adjusting one or two springs. These are a bit more cumbersome than the "single" hand grippers, but go a long way in building grip strength step by step with only one tool.

Before I go into detail with the training for this kind of hand strength, I want to add that hand gripper training has become a real sport recently. Closing a particular gripper is considered by many a feat of strength, and sometimes associated with oldtime strength. However, although closing a very difficult hand gripper is a verifiable, standardised measurement of strength, and a testimony for the great hand strength of an athlete, it cannot really be considered a feat of strength by (my) definition. The appeal of strength feats, in particular for performance purposes, lies in object manipulation. This is most effective when an everyday object is used. For example, if you lift an adult person with your teeth, this is impressive to an audience, as everyone can estimate the weight of a human and imagine the strain on your teeth and jaw this causes. Or, if you tear a deck of 52 cards or more, everyone in the audience can relate to it, as everyone has held a deck of cards in their hands at least once and knows they can tear a playing card easily, but probably not if it is multiplied by 52 – and so on. The same is true of a different discipline in the performing circus arts, which is the work of illusionists and magicians. A magic trick is only truly effective if it is performed with an object everyone in the audience can relate to (to a certain degree). When a magician lets a live rabbit disappear in his hat, everyone will be awestruck. When he manipulates an abstract contraption nobody in the audience has ever seen before, the effect will be much smaller (although some magicians do work in this way).

This also makes feats of strength with barbells, dumbbells, and kettlebells a bit problematic, because only the people in the audience who can test the weight will actually have an idea of the difficulty of the feat. For everyone else, the barbell could be anything from very light to very heavy – one can really not tell simply by looking at it. However, barbells, dumbbells, and kettlebells can almost be considered everyday objects in these days, as training with weights has become increasingly popular (I have also made the experience that audiences particularly enjoy feats with archaic-looking dumbbells and kettlebells, perhaps because this is what they expect to see in an oldtime strongman performance). Still, the large majority of people are not familiar with heavy-duty hand grippers. Thus, you can only impress a small group of experts with the "feat" of closing such a gripper. Keep this in mind: For a performing oldtime strongman, hand gripper training should only be a means to an end, to build stronger hands for more suitable feats of strength.

To illustrate this, consider the best feat of strength in the dynamic hand strength category: crushing a raw potato with one hand. This feat has become timeless and classic through its depiction in the adventure novel *The Sea-Wolf* by the American writer Jack London. In the now famous scene of the novel, the brutish sea captain Wolf Larsen crushes a raw potato in the ship's galley, to demonstrate his animalistic strength to the shipwrecked protagonist Humphrey van Weyden:

> "I was peeling potatoes. He [Wolf Larsen] picked one up from the pan. It was fair-sized, firm, and unpeeled. He closed his hand upon it, squeezed, and the potato squirted out between his fingers in mushy streams. The pulpy remnant he dropped back into the pan and turned away, and I had a sharp vision of how it might have fared with me had the monster put his real strength upon me."

Of course, it is impossible to crush a potato with one hand in the way Jack London imagined it when writing this scene. This is why he put it in the book: to portray Wolf Larsen as otherworldly strong. However, with the proper technique, something similar can be done, and thus the impossible made possible. I will come back to this later.

If you want to make progress in your dynamic grip strength training, the most obvious way would be the following: Take a gripper with adjustable springs, perform your training with it with a common scheme of sets and repetitions in a low range (about three to five), and gradually, step by step, increase the resistance by adjusting the springs. The next possibility would be to work with the single hand grippers I described above, also with a common scheme of repetitions and sets, until you are able to move to the next step of gripper (as the resistance of these cannot be adjusted). However, as mentioned, you will not yet be able to work with the next step of gripper if you can close one particular gripper five times – the upper limit of my suggested repetition range. Therefore, one way of progressing would be to gradually increase the number of repetitions beyond this range, until you can do about 20 easily, and then move on to the next gripper.

Although this method works in principle, it is not a very efficient method. Doing sets of 15 and more repetitions is strength endurance training, more than training for maximum strength. Therefore, I suggest you try a different method of progression, which is the following: Not everyone who starts training with these grippers is aware how much of a difference it makes a) whether the gripper is properly held in one's hand, and b) how far the handles of the gripper are apart at the beginning of the repetition. To take care of a), you should first of all learn how to "set" the gripper in your hand. This you do by pressing the end of one handle deep into the palm of the given hand (with the thumb of the assisting hand), namely in such a manner that it rest against the thumb pad of the given hand. Then, the fingers of the assisting hand pull on the other handle and support the given hand in getting a really good grip on it. In this way, the gripper is already "closed" to a certain degree before you even begin your repetition. This is not considered cheating, as you will only be able to close such a hand gripper if it is properly *set* in your hand. You will soon realize that you can thus use your assisting hand to close the gripper to a larger or smaller degree, however you prefer.

The next aspect that most people are not immediately aware of when they start training with such grippers, is that the farther the handles are apart at the beginning of the movement, the harder the gripper is to close. For example, if the handles are two centimetres apart, the hand gripper will be easier to close than when they are four centimetres apart.

This principle can be applied to your training to have a means for progression. For example: You start training on a particular gripper by always setting it in your hand in such a way that the handles are roughly one centimetre apart. In this manner you do sets of three to five repetitions (by repetition I mean closing the gripper until the handles touch). Once you can easily do more than five repetitions in this manner, you continue your training by setting the gripper in your hand in such a way that the handles are two centimetres apart. Once you can easily do more than five repetitions in this way, you do your repetitions with the handles three centimetres apart, and so on.

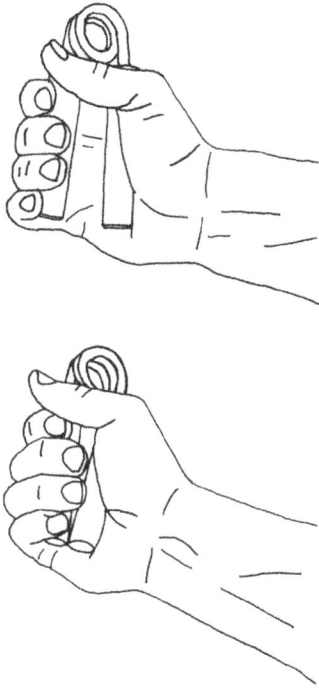

Figure 9.13 Setting a hand gripper (above) and closing a hand gripper (below).

Once you can easily do more than five repetitions with the handles six centimetres apart, you might be ready to move on to the next gripper and start training on this one with the handle half a centimetre apart in the beginning – and so on (these are only very rough figures and no general laws). I hope you understand what I mean. You progress in your gripper training not by endlessly increasing the number of repetitions, but by gradually increasing the distance of the handles in the beginning of the movement, thus making training on the same gripper more difficult. But you always stay in a low repetition level.

There are a few feats of strength that require dynamic, or crushing, strength from the thumbs. One example is crushing a walnut with the thumb, or crushing a can of beer by pushing your thumbs into the metal. Regular hand gripper training does not actively train your thumbs. If you do want to have a reasonably strong thumb, training with thick bar weights and pinch grip training are a good way to go, although these only require static thumb strength. If, by all means possible, you want to train your thumb for dynamic strength, there are a few methods as well. Some companies produce special training equipment for this type of strength, and there are simple ways to rebuild such equipment at home as well (I talk about this in my book *Grip Strength*). Last but not least, you can use a light hand gripper for thumb training as well.

Once you have reached a considerable level of hand strength in one of the three categories above (or two, or all three categories), and want to achieve a particular feat of grip strength, you should start training for the feat itself. If, for example, you trained for some years with hand grippers, i.e. for dynamic grip strength, because one day you want to be able to crush a large, fresh, and raw potato in your hand (crushing a small and foul raw potato in your hand is no feat of strength), you should at some point in time start training with actual potatoes.

The way to do this is to drive your fingertips right into the middle of the potato and then finish it off with a motion like you would close a hand gripper. Imagine using your four fingers like one large, blunt blade to cut the potato in half. Although you are actually halving the potato rather than "crushing" it, it will give a similar impression if you do it fast. Note that the larger the potato and the wider your hand is open, the harder it is going to be.

Even in the training for such a feat there are ways to have progression, although the natural irregularity of fruit and vegetables, like potatoes, makes it rather difficult. As a general rule, I suggest you only train with the same variety of potato and with similar sizes to start with. In the beginning you could also crush potatoes that are partially cooked – for example, having been boiled for ten minutes. Once you can manage these, you continue with potatoes that have been boiled for five minutes, and so on. Please do not forget to wait until they have cooled down, and, if possible, perform your training in a clean environment. Then you can still use the crushed potatoes to make them into a meal of mashed potatoes later on, so that you do not have to waste food.

Likewise, although I also believe in specialization, or *focalization*, when training for a great feat of grip strength, grip strength training also benefits from the principle of *variation*. Although each type of grip strength feat requires specialized training, training for one will eventually contribute to the other types of grip strength feats as well. Also, you can make progress by experimenting with your grip, technique, etc. within your training for one particular type of grip strength feat. The principle of *partialisation* can be applied to grip strength training only to a limited degree, as most grip strength feats do not have the kind of complexity that makes partialisation necessary or possible. That the principle of *continuity* is of utmost importance to grip strength training should be self-explanatory, as a high level of grip strength requires training over very long periods of time.

9.6. Teeth Strength

Teeth strength training and feats have some advantages and some disadvantages. One big advantage is that a) when you perform a teeth strength feat in front of an audience, it is relatively easy to impress, even with a mediocre achievement, because most people do not have a reference of what is possible with teeth strength and what not. Their horizon is somewhat limited, so to say. Lifting a mediocre weight with the teeth, or bending an easy piece of steel in your jaw, are usually sufficient to impress an audience. I am not trying to say that you should be satisfied with a mediocre performance, but what I am trying to say is that teeth strength feats are a relatively simple method to enhance an oldtime strongman show.

Another advantage is that b) biting, and some of the movements that teeth strength feats and their training involve, are quite natural movements for which our body is built, as I have explained earlier. Thus, if you want to train your whole body, there is no real good reason to leave teeth strength out. Not many people are aware of the fact that our jaw muscles are, in relation to their size, the strongest muscles in our body, so why not take advantage of this and develop them even further?

A third advantage is that c) if teeth strength training is natural to our body and our bodies are made for it, it follows that teeth strength training is also *good* for our body. First of all, it is a well-known fact that in certain sports, like boxing, wrestling, and motorcycling, a strong neck is of utmost importance to reduce the risk of serious injury and trauma to the head. While there are a few effective methods to train your neck without the involvement of your teeth, for example with a head harness, why not train for teeth strength and build your neck muscles along the way? In fact – and I will talk more about this later – if your train for a variety of different teeth strength feats, you will train all the important muscles in your neck, which move your head into the various directions it can be moved.

In my opinion (although I do not have scientific proof for it yet), a further health benefit of teeth strength training is that it reduces the risk of some common teeth problems (quite contrary to what one would expect). Everybody knows that our bodies were made to move, rather than remain immobile, and a certain physical stress is beneficial to our bones, muscles, circulatory system, and overall health, when compared to, for example, a purely sedentary lifestyle. The so-called Western civilization tends to *suffer* more and more from an overly *comfortable* (read inactive) lifestyle rather than the other way round. It follows that also our teeth, jaws, etc. work *too little* rather than too much. One could say they enjoy too much *comfort*, which is obvious when we look at the kind of food we, in our society, consider pleasant, tasty, and even sophisticated to eat. A tender piece of steak is considered superior to a piece of meat that is tough like the sole of a shoe.

Some experts believe that one reason why children in Western and Westernized countries have so many problems with malpositioned teeth, and why almost *every* child requires braces at one point in their lives, is because the food they regularly eat is processed too much and therefore too soft. But to grow big and strong, the jawbone requires stress from time to time – just as every other bone in our body. As a consequence, the jaws of children in so-called civilized societies are regularly underdeveloped. The teeth, which cannot alter their size, have too little room and grow irregularly.

I do not want to put my head too far above the parapet, as I am neither a medic nor an oral surgeon or dentist, but I also have the suspicion that underdeveloped jawbones could be a factor that favours the problems so many adults have with their wisdom teeth. These have to be taken out with often very painful and risky surgery on millions of patients every year. The fact that we humans even have wisdom teeth, which usually never surface in the course of our lives, is proof that our jaws are generally becoming smaller and smaller – but this is happening over long time periods and there is hardly a remedy. However, it is a commonly known fact that especially in the last two hundred years, our human culture has evolved at a rapid pace – among other things toward an automated, overproducing, processed-food industry and a more and more inactive lifestyle – and our bodies cannot keep track. This concerns our jaws and teeth just as the rest of our bodies.

Also, not many young people ever spend a thought on the fact why their teeth stay in their mouths from day to day and not simply fall out. They are kept in position by connective tissue. As everybody knows, tendons, bones, muscles, etc. grow strong and stay healthy when regularly stressed, so it would appear logic to me that this connective tissue needs regular stress and training as well. But this is just my observation and opinion, and you should not prefer this to professional medical advice. There are lots of factors that influence the health of our teeth and mouths, in particular bacteria, which can dissolve teeth, gums, etc. and cause inflammations, regardless of the stress and training they receive.

This already leads me to the disadvantages of teeth strength training. One minor problem is that a) teeth strength training is considered odd and exotic, and people might consider you a "freak" when they see you trying feats of teeth strength. Therefore, you might not feel comfortable doing such in the company of others.

However, the biggest disadvantages of teeth strength training, and the reason why most people never try it, are b) the (health) risks involved. In the perception of most people, these risks outweigh the health advantages, and one can certainly say that if your teeth strength training, or feats, do go wrong, the damage is potentially greater than all the benefits. These risks obviously contain that you might damage one or several of your teeth – in the best case by losing them, in the worst case by breaking them.

If you lose a complete tooth, or if it becomes loose in the course of a teeth strength feat gone wrong, there is a chance that a dentist or oral surgeon will be able to put it back into place or that it will even grow back on by itself (this has once happened to the oldtime strongman and personal friend of mine Rainer Schröder from Thuringia).

If you break a tooth, however, there is nothing in the world that can make it whole again. Other than our bones, muscles, and even ligaments, our teeth have no potential to repair themselves. Although surgeons and dentists in our days can *repair* most of this kind of damage, your actual tooth will be gone or damaged forever, for the rest of your life. I know several oldtime strongman and circus artists who have lost a tooth, or part of a tooth, in the course of teeth strength feats.

This is the biggest risk that one who plans to try teeth strength training and feats should always keep in mind (this being said, there are some sports that I consider much more dangerous to your teeth, like ice hockey). Some teeth strength feats also put a great stress on your cervical spine, which is a risk of a very different kind and not to be underestimated by any means.

Now that I have talked of the benefits and risks of teeth strength training, let me talk about some of the different feats of strength that can be done with the teeth and jaw, and how to train for them. Also teeth strength feats can be grouped into categories:

1. Lifting feats
2. Towing feats
3. Bending feats
4. Balancing and supporting feats

Ad 1): *Lifting feats* are the most obvious and straightforward teeth strength feats, although they can be as varied as the objects lifted. A classic feat is lifting a person from the floor, and this always works well in front of an audience, because you can use someone from the audience as the weight. Mind you that lifting feats put an outward-pulling stress on your teeth and jaw on an imaginary horizontal line when you stand upright. This is quite a natural stress on your teeth, and it the same stress prehistoric men and women who tanned leather by holding it in their mouths experienced. The straight muscles on the back of our necks, which are most stressed in this feat, are by nature quite strong and potent. However, as most teeth lifting feats are done while standing, and in a bent-over manner, they put a great stress on your cervical spine. If the weight is heavy enough, this can cause you to assume a very unnatural and risky posture.

To perform any kind of teeth lifting feat, one needs a mouthpiece to which the weight is attached. This is the biggest secret to teeth lifting feats, as only a proper mouthpiece enables you to lift heavy weights with your teeth. This being said, such mouthpieces come in all shapes and sizes, and there is no general rule regarding material, mechanics, or looks. I use a leather mouthpiece, as I prefer natural materials whenever possible. It consists of a piece of sturdy leather, cut to something resembling a dumbbell-shape, and folded once, to make a double layer. The sling caused by this fold is where I attach the weight to with the help of a large shackle. The doubled up part is cut to the shape of my mouth, which I did in the following way: I took a piece of cardboard, bit into it, and used the impression of my teeth as a stencil for the leather. I addition to this, I took two pieces of leather, shaped to the inside of my upper and lower row of teeth, and put them on the top and bottom of the leather piece. Then I fastened everything together with a screw really tightly. This screw has to be retightened every once in a while. I clean my leather mouthpiece regularly with a toothbrush, and maintain it with a hundred per cent natural beeswax balm I make myself.

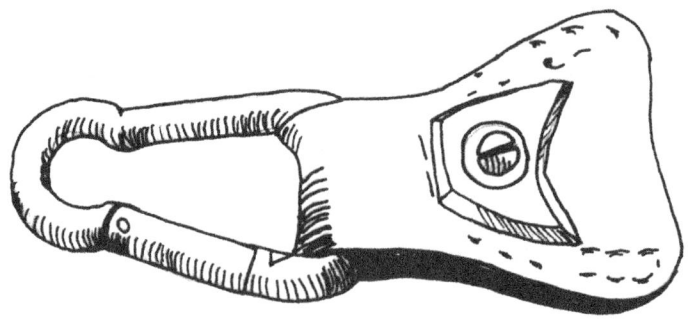

Figure 9.14 My leather mouthpiece.

Such a mouthpiece, if well maintained, lasts for several years of heavy lifting before it has to be replaced. In essence, I modelled my mouthpiece after an old illustration and based on a description in the book *Feats of Strength and Dexterity* by Charles MacMahon. It has the advantage that all the teeth in your mouth have their place on it and can contribute to the lift. The strongest and most essential teeth in this lift are your back teeth, but the leather pieces on the top and bottom push against your front teeth as well, adding a few additional kilograms you will be able to lift.

Every oldtime strongman has his mouthpiece of preference. I know one person who has a similar mouthpiece, but it is not folded up. Instead, it consists of one large, very thick piece of leather with a hole at the bottom to which the weight is attached. Also, it puts most of the stress on the front teeth, which I do not prefer, but it works for him. I also know someone who uses simply a sturdy piece of cloth he doubles up to cause a sling, and a piece of leather he puts between it (shaped to his mouth). It works stunningly well for him.

Then, there are the types of mouthpieces circus artists use, which have a steel core and a cast of their individuals mouths of artificial, non-elastic material. These must be custom-made by an expert, like a dentist, and probably have the highest potency. They function like a clamp in your mouth where your teeth and the mouthpiece have no way to go. The kinds of feats some circus artists (men and women) perform with these are awe-inspiring, and probably exceed some of the simple teeth lifts of some oldtime strongmen by far. However, I do not want to know what would happen if such a mouthpiece, or the teeth, ever gave in under the great stress. I have a mouthpiece like this, custom-made, but do not really like to use it.

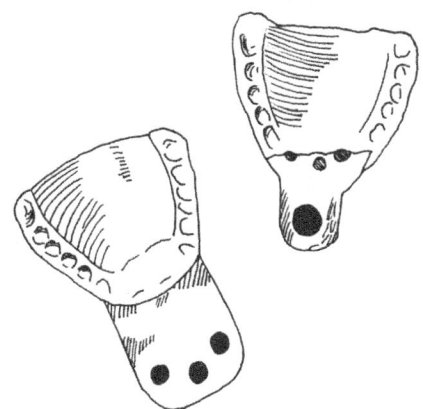

Figure 9.15 Mouthpieces of artificial material.

Whatever type of material or shape you use (perhaps you will come up with your own creative idea of how to construct your mouthpiece), here are two more pieces of advice: a) Use a material that is not poisonous or toxic, so that there are no health concerns when you put it in your mouth. b) When your mouthpiece, as well as the shackle you use, looks big, strong, and hefty, it will add some effect to your lift, as people automatically associate it with a heavier load.

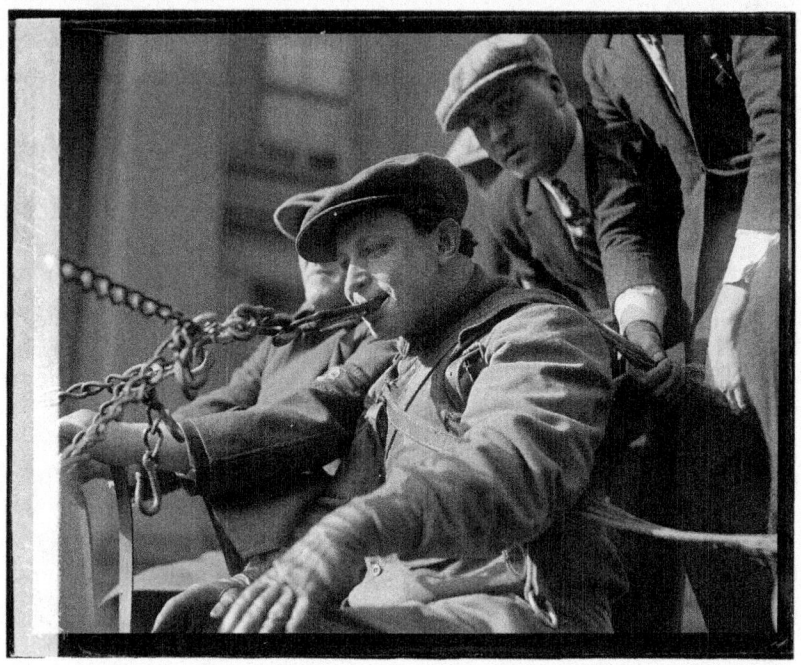

Figure 9.16 The famous strongman Siegmund Breitbart getting ready for a towing feat. The hefty chains and mouthpiece suggest a heavy load.

Once you have found a mouthpiece that works for you, nothing is simpler than training for teeth lifts. All you have to do is find a way to attach weight to your mouthpiece and to increase this weight in small steps. In the beginning, this can be a simple bucket, or a piece of rope that runs through a couple of weight plates. Then, you train the lift with a simple scheme of sets and repetitions, like any other weightlifting exercise. In this way, you can practically start from zero, lifting only a couple of kilograms in the beginning to get a feel. Soon you will realize that a teeth lift is like any other weightlifting exercise, not much different from a deadlift or a bench press. Any lift where you lift the weight clearly off the floor can be considered a good lift – there is no other general rule.

Ad 2): You will need a similar mouthpiece for *towing feats* as for lifting feats. In our days, the object to tow will probably be n automobile, a small bus, or a truck. The first thing you will realize if you ever try this feat, is actually how easy it is to tow a modern automobile with the teeth on a smooth, horizontal surface. I have towed three automobiles in a row in this manner, but I have also towed a creaky horse cart with a musical band on it without much effort. Therefore, this feat only gets interesting once you tow a really big truck or bus, and even so I would argue that the weak link will not be your teeth and jaw, but either your inferior body weight or the traction of your shoes. Towing feats have the advantage over lifting feats that the stress on the cervical spine is smaller and less risky, because you are not in a bent-over position. In fact, they feel quite pleasant. Also, teeth towing feats are popular and always cause a little sensation. They can be performed practically anywhere where enough space, a safe environment, and vehicles to tow are around.

Ad 3): *Bending feats* belong to the more risky teeth strength feats. Of course, the risk depends on the degree of difficulty, and one can always use soft enough steel to reduce the risk to a tolerable degree. With some training, however, it is possible to bend very tough steel with the help of your teeth and jaw, making for very impressive and show-proof feats of strength. Thus, I have seen anything from steel bars, nails, horseshoes, to coins being bent with the help of the teeth. The interesting aspect is that the variety of teeth strength feats that is known makes it possible to train your jaw and neck from a great variety of angles and into various directions – forward, backward, sideways, in a twisting motion, and so on.

The most straightforward and classic teeth strength steel bending feat is bending a round steel bar with the help of your jaw. It is very simple, because all you will need is a lengthy steel bar and some padding. Wrap the padding (preferably leather) around the centre of the bar. Then you practically bite into the centre of the bar, but actually push it as far back into the jaw as possible, so that it rests on your back teeth. Next, you grab the ends of the bar with your hands. Most of the times, and especially in the beginning, you will not need pads for your hands, because the weak link of the feat will be your teeth strength. As you progress to shorter and tougher bars, you might eventually need padding for your hands as well. Then you simply pull down on the ends of the bar until it is reasonably bent, take it out of your mouth, and continue the bend until the ends of the bar are parallel to each other (which is when the bar can be considered fully bent), or you bend it to parallel while holding it in your mouth. In

111

fact, your teeth and jaw will only be stressed during the beginning of this movement, but not after the bar is already considerably bent. By then, your mouth will not function as much more than a stabilizer.

In sum, this feat is the same as bending a long steel bar in any other braced bending technique – whether against your thigh, knee, neck, or head. That you hold the bar in your mouth only differentiates this technique from others by the fact that it looks spectacular to an audience, and – unfortunately – that it is not suitable for extremely tough steel bars. First of all, the position of your hands and especially elbows in relation to your mouth are not ideal to exert maximum force, and secondly, your jaw can never offer the kind of resistance against the downward pulling movement of your hands as, for example, your thigh. Nevertheless, it is a nice act. In a similar manner, also short steel can be bent when the teeth hold *one* end of the steel, like nails, horseshoes, etc. But you will never able to bend the same kind of steel as you could with the usual bending technique for these feats.

There might be one exception, which are coins. It seems that American one-cent coins, or pennies, belong to the rare specimens of coins that can theoretically be bent with hands only, although I have only heard of two strongmen, "Stanless Steel" and Chris "Hairculese" Rider, both from America, who are able to do this. Tommy Heslep, who is known for his grip strength, is able to bend an American ten-cent coin, or dime, with the help of his teeth in the following manner: He holds one half of the coin with his back teeth (with the help of some leather padding – you should never ever try steel bending feats with steel against teeth only), and pushes against the other half with his thumb. In this manner, he is able to cause a visible bend in the coin. It is Mr Heslep's great thumb strength that assists him in this feat, and perhaps it is really the thumb that is the weak link here, rather than the teeth.

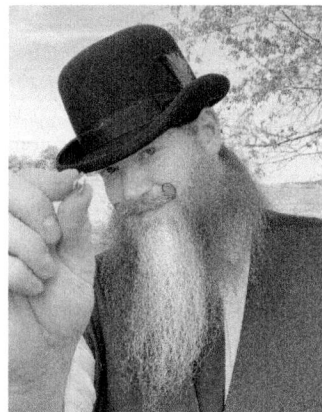

Figure 9.17 Strongman Chris "Hairculese" Rider with one-cent coin he has bent.

The situation changes somewhat, as soon as you make use of a vice, which can increase the leverage tremendously. Once you clamp one end of any piece of steel in a vice that is fixed to a sturdy table or work bench, and bend it with the help of your jaw by biting onto the other end, you will be able to bend very tough objects. My friend Rainer Schröder from Germany is the expert in these kinds of feats and has bent very tough horseshoes, wrenches, and coins (typically a one-Euro-coin) in this manner. Georges Christen from Luxembourg regularly bends and breaks three nails at once with a vice.

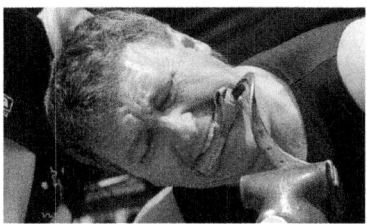

Figure 9.18 Strongman Rainer Schröder bending a horseshoe with his teeth.

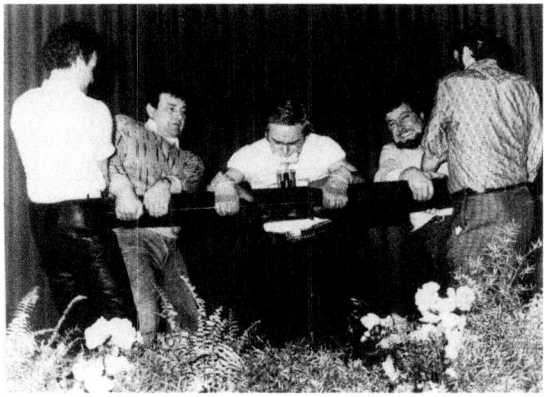

Figure 9.19 Strongman Georges Christen bending three nails with his teeth.

The training for these kinds of feats is not much different from other steel bending feats, and you progress by starting with light steel and experimenting with padding and technique. The two particularities of teeth strength steel bending feats are only that they are risky (and, as a direct consequence, great for show purposes) and that there will be a lot more experimenting with technique necessary. In general, though, once you try such a feat with a light piece of steel, you will be surprised how easy it actually is, and how much it is the fear of getting hurt that limits you, rather than the tremendous natural power of your jaw.

113

Ad 4): There exist some absolutely stunning *balancing and supporting feats* that utilize teeth strength, but the most amazing ones actually belong to the field of circus acrobatics, more than to the field of the oldtime strongman – by tradition, by the way they are staged, and by the way they incorporate other skills, like balancing and acrobatic ability. Within the circus disciplines, the transition is fluent from very light balancing feats, for example, where the artist balances a sword or the like on a dagger she holds in her mouth, with which she then climbs ladders, etc., to such stunts like the one where an acrobat balances on a device that another acrobat holds in his jaws with a mouthpiece.

Some of these feats are obviously much more impressive than the things some oldtime strongmen do and have done. However, they are staged in a very different manner, emphasising aesthetics rather than raw strength and power, and emphasising the act rather than the physicality of the athlete. Therefore, again, they should be put in a different category: the acrobatic category, which is, in my perception, more about *the inversion of physical laws*, in contrast to the strongman category, which is more about *making the impossible possible* – although the two are obviously related.

The same is true, by the way, of acrobatic feats that are similar to teeth lifting feats, but are part of an acrobatic circus performance, like supporting an acrobat from a trapeze by a mouthpiece, or the roller-skate stunt where one acrobat holds the other by a mouthpiece while doing fast pirouettes on a tiny platform.

Because of the existence of such feats, it is questionable whether an oldtime strongman should even touch upon teeth balancing and supporting feats. He will never be able to perform equally stunning feats as some circus artists without the proper acrobatic background. One must also not forget that oldtime strongmen have practically died out within the traditional circus, with some very rare exceptions (which are very popular with audiences!). The perfection of stunts like the above by circus acrobats – stunts that combine agility, acrobatic skill *and* great strength – might be partly responsible for having made the figure of the circus strongman obsolete. Therefore, a modern circus *strongman* will probably have to find a niche that differentiates him from the circus *acrobat*, and stage feats of raw, unsophisticated, momentary, and maximum strength across short ranges of motion, with a deliberate negation of the need for aesthetics that the circus has more and more made its defining asset.

This being said, I nevertheless want to talk about three teeth supporting/balancing feats I have successfully incorporated into my show. These are a chair balancing feat, a table supporting feat, and a barrel supporting feat. You already realize that all of these feats incorporate everyday objects, which is always the best premise for an oldtime strongman feat.

114

The chair feat is about balancing a chair with a person sitting on it on your head, or jaw, however you want to put it. Because in actual fact, you *stabilize* the chair with your jaw by biting into the back stretcher (the horizontal piece of wood that connects the rear legs), and *balance* about two thirds of the weight on your forehead. Thus, the feat does several interesting things: a) It takes an ordinary object and an ordinary situation (a person sitting on a chair), but takes it out of its ordinary context (the person with chair hovers above the heads of the audience). b) It creates the illusion, or "script" that you are holding the chair with your teeth, because the audience perceives how you bite into the rung of the chair, although the larger percentage of the weight is balanced on your forehead (where any human can in theory support very large loads). More on the term "script" later. c) It creates a feeling of danger, because teeth strength *and* height are involved.

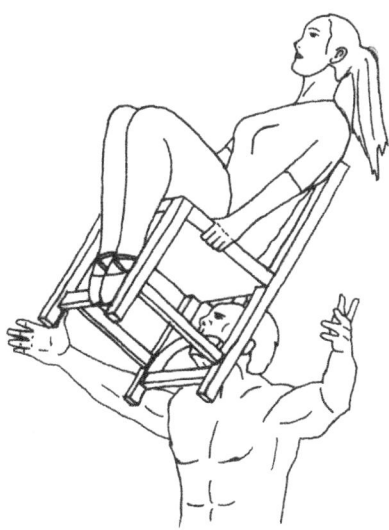

Figure 9.20 The chair balancing feat.

In sum, the chair balancing feat is a beautiful feat of teeth strength that is impressing without any knowledge of the exact weight that is manipulated. It goes without saying that the skill of the assistant, the person sitting on the chair, can make all the difference in this feat. Although I have lifted relatively heavy and completely unprepared volunteers from the audience in this manner, mind you that the worst thing that can happen to you as a performing artist is when someone from your audience gets hurt through your fault.

Also, the amount of balancing skill and bravery of your assistant can make the feat more difficult or easier, regardless of the body weight of the person. Not everyone is aware of this, but in the course of my acrobatic training I realized that an assistant who knows how to maintain body tension can be much easier to lift that a lighter person with no acrobatic experience. Therefore, ideally, you can train and perform the feat with an assistant of your choice. The chair balancing feat is a nice contrast to most teeth lifting and towing feats, as it puts stress on your jaw in an *inward* and *downward* direction.

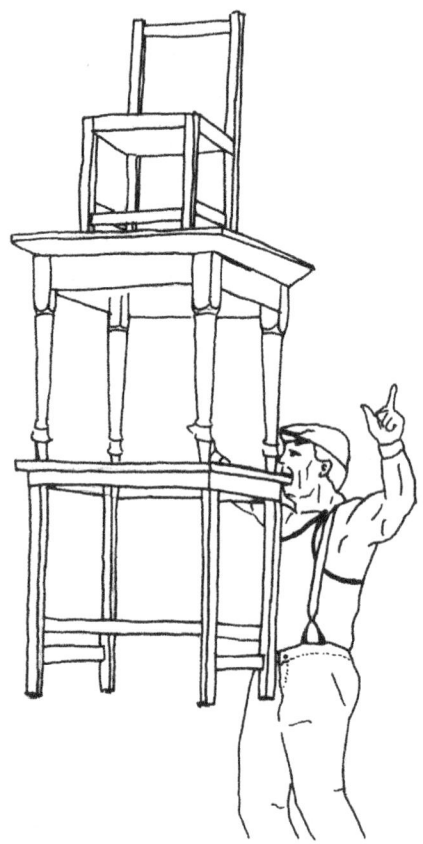

Figure 9.21 The table supporting feat.

The table supporting feat uses a similar principle as the chair balancing feat, but it is performed with a table instead of a chair. This has the advantage that a table is, in the minds of the audience, heavier than a chair. It can be performed with an assistant or without. If you perform the feat without an assistant, it creates the best image if you use a quadrangular table.

The way to perform it is the following: You bite into one of the corners of the quadrangular table and lift it in such a manner that the leg of the table on this corner rests against your chest and abdomen, and the table top remains parallel to the ground. The feat creates a nice image and is made easier by the fact that the leg resting against your chest takes some of the load away from your mouth. In this manner, a man with reasonably strong teeth can lift any small quadrangular table of wood, if he does not mind biting into the corner of it. If you do not want to ruin the table, mind you that your teeth will probably leave traces in the wood. The feat can be performed with several tables on top of each other, making for a magnificent visual image – high and perceptible from afar. If the table is sturdy enough, it can also be performed with one table but with a child sitting on it.

If you want to use a heavier assistant than a child, there is a more efficient variation to the feat. Georges Christen regularly demonstrates it in his show (he has even set a world record in this feat). In this variation, you use a slightly rectangular table and bite into one of the long edges of the table top, rather than into the corner. The assistant sits on the table top, but slides far back, so that she sits very close to the mouth of the strongman. The "trick" in this variation is that the table must have a bottom stretcher (like the chair in the chair feat), which rests against the abdomen of the strongman, like the leg of the table in the first variation. This makes the feat easier, or rather possible, but still difficult enough.

In the context of this feat, Georges Christen has pointed out an interesting fact to me with regard to performance psychology. He always asks for a volunteer lady from the audience weighing no more than 50kg (110lbs). In this manner he makes sure that an assistance steps forward who has a maximum weight of *60kg* (132lbs). This is because confident people are a bit lenient with, or ignorant of, their own body weight. One should always take this into consideration when incorporating people from the audience.

This being said, the feat is obviously easier to train and perform if you use an assistant you are used to and have trained the feat with. Any variation of the table feat stresses the mouth and jaw in an *outward* (like in a regular teeth lift or tow) and slightly *downward* direction.

The barrel supporting feat has the advantage that it incorporates an interesting everyday object – a large barrel – but it has the disadvantage that it requires a mouthpiece, like in any teeth lifting or towing feat. This mouthpiece needs to be attached to the rim of one end of the barrel. The barrel itself can be heavy or light. This does not matter so much, as the challenge should always be the weight of an assistant sitting on the barrel. Of course, if the barrel itself is heavy as well, the feat is more impressive.

The way to perform it is the following: The barrel should rest on a high table, so that the mouthpiece is at a height slightly below your mouth. Then, your assistant or assistants sit down on the barrel, much like on a horse. It is an advantage if the assistant can somehow hold on to the barrel, for example on the front rim. Take care that the assistant does not sit too close to your mouthpiece, because otherwise the stress will be too much in a downward direction rather than in a forward direction, which it should be (like in a teeth lift or tow). Then, maybe with the help of your hands to stabilize the barrel, you lift the load up (letting the bottom of the barrel rest against your chest like in the table lifting feats above) and, once everything is stable, let go with your hands, to demonstrate that you support the barrel and assistant with your teeth only (and chest, of course).

Success in training for any such teeth balancing or supporting feats lies particularly in two aspects: a) the equipment (or props), and b) the principle of progression. As to a), the equipment has to be just right. You cannot perform the chair balancing feat with a chair that has no back stretcher. Also, the feat will not be successful if the chair breaks the moment your balance it on your forehead. The barrel feat will not work and have no effect if the barrel is too small – and so on. Thus, you can only start training for such feats once you have the proper equipment. This might mean that you will have to construct parts of it yourself, or have them custom-made. Then there is always the risk that custom-made props will be useless, because of some aspect you did not take into consideration (for example, if the back stretcher of the chair is too low).

Once you do have the ideal equipment, how do you b) progress in feats of strength that use an assistant? First of all, before you start training for these slightly more complex feats, you should already have developed some basic teeth strength by teeth lifting training.

Next, smaller assistants are obviously easier to lift, but they cannot be endlessly small. In addition to this, you should never *start* training for a risky feat of strength with *children,* as you do not want them to get hurt. So what you do is, you use sandbags as weights and fix them to your props with ratchet straps. Purchase 25kg (55lbs) sandbags, or fill any bag with the amount of weight of sand you need. In this way you can comfortably train such feats of strength without live persons until you have mastered a considerable load. Once you can perform them in training with 50kg (110lbs) of weight in sandbags, you can start training with a grown-up assistant who (really) weighs 50kg (110lbs).

Mind you that the weight is distributed differently if you use a live person rather than sandbags. You assistant should be very well instructed, have some acrobatic experience, trust you, and be fearless. In every other case you add unnecessary risk. Only once you are absolutely sure you can do the feat easily with a grown-up person of 50kg (110lbs) and more, should you start thinking about doing it with volunteers from an audience.

9.7. (Kettlebell) Juggling

Juggling is a separate discipline within the circus arts, and one could argue that good jugglers who do nothing else (and have done nothing else for many years) have such a high skill level that aspiring oldtime strongmen would be well-advised to stay away from juggling. Still, I would argue that juggling with *heavy objects* is still a discipline reserved for the strongman. Then, juggling has all the advantages for the strongman that it has for any performing juggler: It is beautiful, it is rhythmic, it is amazing, it can be repeated endlessly, and it is healthy (the latter is only true of juggling heavy weights if you do not drop them on your head or toes).

The wonderful Cirque du Soleil production *Alegría* featured different oldtime strongmen, and one of these, Stepan Ivanov, regularly performed a teeth lift with ten kettlebells. I will talk a little bit about this in the chapter "Performing". Here I would like to mention that before Stepan Ivanov lifted the kettlebells in this manner, he took two of them, quite casually, and juggled them for less than half a minute, with some very simple movements. But how beautiful this short sequence was! The movements were perfect, it seemed heavy yet easy, and it was an image that had "oldtime strongman" written on it.

But to leave the performance aspect aside for the moment, kettlebell juggling is a wonderful exercise in itself. Whether done for an audience or not, it practices strength, speed, coordination, responsiveness, and strength endurance at the same time (if done properly).

However, I do not want to add fuel to the fire of the recent hype that praises this traditional training equipment beyond all measures. It has its disadvantages as well. For example, you will need an extra set of kettlebells for any step of progression you make. Also, many modern kettlebells are quite ugly and constructed of artificial material that cannot be repaired when broken. Even some of the modern kettlebells of metal are of inferior quality and break easily. To counter these problems, I strongly recommend you wait with the purchase of kettlebells until you are a hundred per cent sure that the right moment has come. Then, for the time being, I would only invest in *one* kettlebell of superior quality, with a weight that can *really* be utilized for purposeful training. What I mean is, it should not be too lightweight. Of course it should be of metal and, ideally, it should be welded, not cast. Such a kettlebell will obviously be more expensive, but more worth the money than a cheaper one.

The best way to train with kettlebells is outdoors, in the fresh air, where there is no risk of breaking the floor. Next, you should decide what you want to do with it. In my opinion there are three uses of a kettlebell for an oldtime strongman: as a warm-up, as an additional weight for a combined feat of strength, or for juggling. I am not so fond of endless repetitions of kettlebell swings or cleans, and I believe they belong more into the type of conditioning training necessary for other sports, like martial arts. The uses of kettlebells for a warm-up and as additional weights are self-explanatory. Thus, if you do regular kettlebell training, the only possibility that is left is juggling.

The whole idea about kettlebell juggling is that the kettlebell is heavy. Therefore, it is acceptable if the juggling movements are simplistic. The heavier the kettlebell, the simpler the movements can be to still constitute a proper feat. A simple *turn* of an 80kg (177lbs) kettlebell is an amazing feat of strength. If your kettlebell is lighter than that (which I suppose), you have lots of other movement possibilities. You can combine these in creative ways to compose a nice juggling routine. Beyond this, you have the possibility to juggle with two kettlebells instead of one. This expands the scope of combinations even further.

Here are some typical kettlebell juggling moves. The names I gave them are purely my invention – I do not know if any kettlebell specialists of aficionados have other, standardized names for them:

- *The forward flip:* This is the most basic kettlebell juggling move. You start with a simple kettlebell swing forward, let go of the handle, and the bell, taking up this momentum, rotates forward freely, until you catch it again by the handle after a full rotation of 360 degrees on a horizontal axis.

- *The backward flip:* Similar to the forward flip, but here you make the bell consciously rotate *backwards*, by giving it a deliberate thrust in the opposite direction than in which it would naturally rotate. After a full rotation of 360 degrees on a horizontal axis you catch it by the handle, which comes up from the bottom.

- *The sideward flip:* This is done in a similar manner as the two movements above, but shortly before you let go of the bell you turn the handle by ninety degrees, so that it is already vertical while you still hold onto it. Then you give it a sideward thrust just before you let it go, either to the left or to the right. The bell should then rotate by 360 degrees on a *vertical axis*, before you catch it again by the handle (which should be vertical throughout the rotation). This can also be done without turning the handle by 90 degrees, and by leaving it horizontal, but this is less beautiful.

- *The hand switch:* All of these flipping movement can also be started with one hand and finished with the other, i.e. one hand starts the rotation and the other hand catches the bell afterwards.

- *The double flip:* All of the flips above are rather simple and easy movements, but where it starts to become interesting, are double flips (of all of these), i.e. making the bell rotate twice by 360 degrees. It takes quite an amount of coordinative skill and practice to do this, even with a simple forward flip. As you practice, the kettlebell will probably drop on the floor quite often. There is also a risk of getting hurt. So practice cautiously.

- *The clock turn:* This is a rather simple movement, where you give the bell a thrust in a (counter-) clockwise motion from your wrist, as if winding up an alarm clock or turning a key in a lock. It will make the handle turn in a (counter-) clockwise motion in front of your eyes, by 180, 360, or more degrees.

- *The overhead catch:* In this beautiful trick, you catch the bottom of the kettlebell above your head on your stretched arm. You do a long and high swing with your fully stretched arm, almost a snatch, but let go of the handle shortly before your arm points fully upward. You let the kettlebell take up the momentum and rotate backward, like in a backward flip, but only by circa 180 degrees, and make it land with its bottom on the palm of your hand, on your fully stretched, upward pointing arm. This movement looks terrific, but please bear in mind the risk involved. In the worst-case scenario, a missed kettlebell could drop onto your head. An intermediate step towards this feat would be to make the bell only turn circa 90 degrees and catch it by its front, so that the handle points forward.

- *The overhead hand switch:* To end the overhead catch, you could simply reverse the movement by giving the kettlebell a slight thrust into a forward and upward direction, catching it by the handle after a 180 degree turn, and swinging it back down. However, once you are already balancing the kettlebell overhead, you can give it a slight upward thrust, coming from your legs, and quickly catch it on your other, outstretched arm overhead, without the bell really changing its position. In theory, this is also possible with a full flip of the kettlebell, but very difficult and risky.

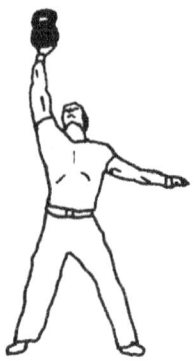

Figure 9.22 The overhead catch.

◆ *The overhead crossing flip:* This movement is also risky, but belongs to the more impressive ones. It involves a turn of your own person by 180 degrees and catching the kettlebell "behind your back", so to say. In essence, you swing the bell high up into the air, above your head and even back slightly, so that it also rotates, like in a backward flip. While it is in the air, you quickly turn by 180 degrees and catch the bell as it comes down, like in a regular backward flip. I hope you can see the coordinative skill and risk involved.

These are just some basic movements and there are countless more. But even these simple movements become exceedingly difficult if, for example, you do double flips instead of single ones, or if you use a heavy kettlebell. Also, they become much more difficult and attractive if you use *two* kettlebells instead of one (where this is possible). Then you also have the possibility to make the two bells switch hands simultaneously, combined with flips, which gets closer to the idea common people have of the word "juggling".

My suggestion is that you try these different moves a little bit, experiment with them, exercise them individually, and eventually put together a routine that you regularly train and try to expand and perfect. Eventually, your progression will lie in smoother movements and transitions, and a more and more elegant execution of the tricks. The more often you train this routine, the more it will enter into your system, until you can practically do it "while you sleep". The thing with juggling is that it is not enough if you *can* do it. You should also be able to do it gracefully. This differentiates juggling from most feats of strength where the *form* is not important, only the fact that you succeed in the feat.

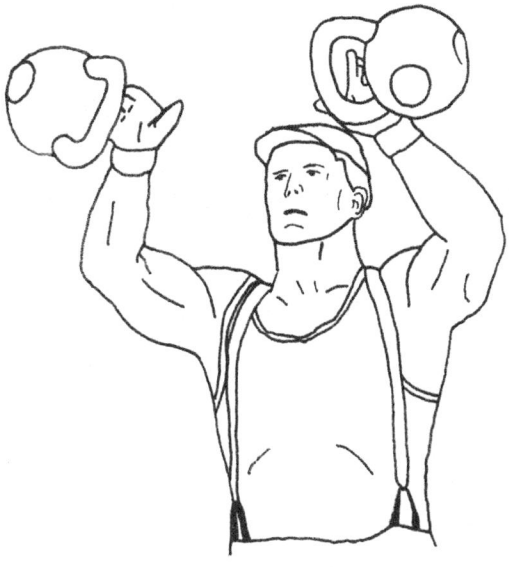

Figure 9.23 A sideward flip with two kettlebells.

Whether you train your kettlebell juggling routine simply for yourself, or for show purposes, the beauty of it is that it belongs to the basic human movement pattern of throwing, mostly replicating the movement of throwing an object *upwards*. It is therefore a welcomed addition and variation to any heavy "throwing" training that only consists of bench press and shoulder press movements. Kettlebell juggling is a great workout for the shoulders, and also puts some stress on back, thighs, hips, and grip. It can therefore never hurt to make kettlebell *juggling* a fixed part of your training regimen (rather than endless swings and cleans with kettlebells, which do not have any real benefit except that they help passing time).

If you have ever considered doing a strongman performance, I should say that there is nothing that beats a proper juggling feat with heavy objects. It is clearly a strongman discipline, yet demonstrates additional coordinative skill that goes beyond pure and raw maximum strength. Apart from kettlebell juggling, you also have the option of doing a "proper" juggling feat. All you need to be able to do is juggle with three objects, for example balls or clubs. This is a skill you have to learn. Then, you progress to heavier and more cumbersome everyday objects. Juggling three iron balls of 10kg (22lbs) each, for example, is a wonderful feat of strength, but it is even better if you use three objects everyone is familiar with and knows as being heavy. Then, nothing can top the beauty of such a feat. My colleague, the Canadian oldtime strongman Mighty Mike (a student of Dennis Rogers), demonstrates this with his feat of juggling a sledgehammer and two torches, or three bowling balls.

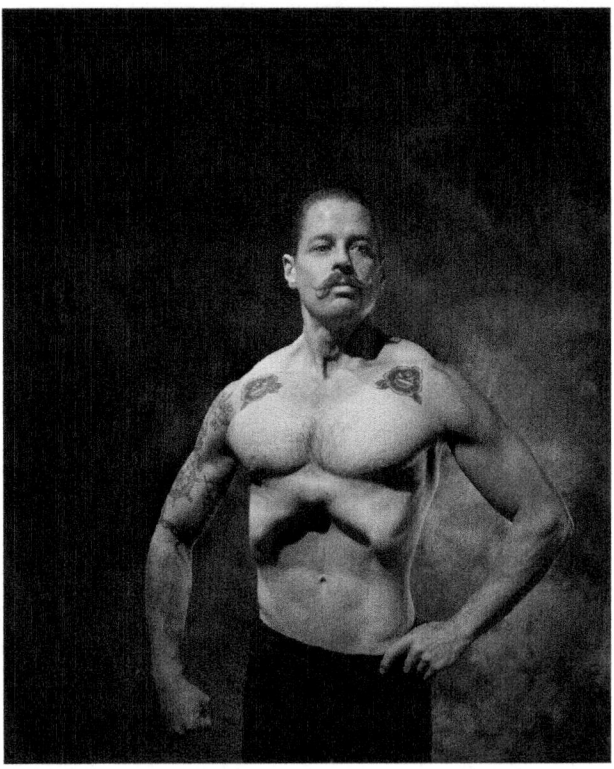

Figure 9.24 Strongman Mighty Mike from Canada.

10. Setting priorities

Above, in the chapter "Feats of strength: Finding your calling", I talked about how to search for your particular area of expertise, or the specific oldtime strongman feats you want to excel at. But there is another kind of specialization, or rather focalization, more in a short-term sense, which you should consider if you want to conquer a feat of strength. Especially if it is a goal very difficult to reach, you will make better progress if you adapt your whole workout routine to the training for this particular feat.

I will demonstrate what I mean by a negative example. Let us recall the amount of possibilities one has to train his body with resistance training. There are seven basic human movement patterns one should cover:

1. Walking, running, and jumping
2. Throwing
3. Climbing
4. Lifting and carrying
5. Hitting
6. Biting
7. Dexterity

For each of these, lots of different weight training exercises with regular barbells, dumbbells, machines, kettlebells, bodyweight, etc. are available. Then, there are several different feats of strength for each movement pattern, as I have shown above. Beyond this, there are further, advanced movement patterns, and if you want to become the ideal athlete, you might want to train some of these as well on some other day of the week:

1. Wrestling
2. Boxing
3. Shooting
4. Horse riding
5. Swimming
6. Paddling
7. Dancing

Based on this, let us assume you have put together a simple workout routine you want to follow each week. You have just started with oldtime strongman training, you are ambitious, and want to become a versatile athlete. You have not found your "calling" yet and want to try as many feats of strength as possible, to get better at each simultaneously. You are already in your late twenties and do not have much time left to become a great oldtime strongman. You have already been to a number of power-lifting meets and plan to attend more, so you also want to improve your squat, bench press, and deadlift – also because you read somewhere that someone who does not squat is not a serious athlete. In addition to this, you want to improve your looks. You want to look stronger as you grow stronger, so you have included some biceps and triceps exercises as well. For the same reason, you put yourself on a diet, because you want to burn a little bit of body fat. This is your workout routine:

Monday (walking, running, jumping):
- ♦ Squats
- ♦ Lunges
- ♦ Leg curl
- ♦ Harness lift

Tuesday (throwing):
- ♦ Bench press
- ♦ Military shoulder press
- ♦ Barbell push press
- ♦ One-arm push press
- ♦ Tricep extension
- ♦ Kettlebell juggling
- ♦ Steel bending

Wednesday (biting):
- ♦ Wrestler's bridges
- ♦ Teeth lift

Thursday (lifting):
- ♦ Deadlifts
- ♦ Stiff-legged deadlifts
- ♦ Barbell rows
- ♦ Thick bar deadlifts
- ♦ One-finger lift
- ♦ Stone lifting (heavy stone)
- ♦ Stone carry (lighter stone)

Friday (dexterity and climbing):
- Pull-ups
- Pull-ups on finger tips
- Pinch lift
- Hand gripper training
- Biceps curl
- Forearm curl
- Reverse forearm curl
- Sledgehammer levering
- Nail bending

Saturday (hitting/swimming and dancing):
- Swimming in the morning
- Sit-ups
- Sledgehammer swings
- Dancing in the evening with spouse

Sunday:
- Rest day

Now this looks like a very ambitious workout plan. Thank God you have a rest day on Sunday. Your spouse will also be grateful that you take some time off for her on Saturday evenings, while you dedicate all the other evenings to improving yourself and becoming that great, swelled-chested athlete.

Let me tell you that this is not an approach I recommend. First of all, training six days a week with great intensity is rather ambitious, and only possible if you are young. Secondly, you are trying to dance at several weddings at the same time, as we say in German (and I do not mean the Saturday evenings). Becoming great at all these feats of strength at the same time, while doing heavy basic exercises like the squat, bench press, and deadlift, and training for looks, and all of this while you are on a diet, will simply not yield the results you hope for. At least in one of these areas, but probably in several of them, your performance will stagnate, or become worse. It is questionable whether you will make any progress worth mentioning in any of these areas at all.

I recommend a different approach. Try to *focus* on only one, or, at the most, two or three goals at the same time. A goal can be, for example, a powerlifting meet, increased muscle size, reduced body fat, or a certain feat of strength. You already realize that only the last of these has specifically to do with oldtime strongman training. So if this is your pick (and I hope it will be, because why else would you be reading this book), the feat of strength might be, for example, a grip strength, teeth strength, steel-bending, or lifting feat.

Let us assume your pick is a steel-bending feat. Then you can still choose between nail bending, steel-bar bending, horseshoe bending, etc. You have all of these options and more – so it would be wise if you made a choice and then focused on it. Of course, you do not have to focus on one feat forever. You can change the focus once you have reached a certain goal, or once you realize this feat is not for you, or simply after half a year. But do make a choice in the beginning and stick to it for a considerable time. Do not try to get better at three weightlifting exercises and six feats of strength at the same time. Do not change your focus every two weeks. Do not go on a diet and start training for a new feat of strength – if you want to become stronger, eat properly. Simply do one thing at a time, focus, and channel your energy. As Benjamin Franklin said, "Let each part of your business have its time."

I have, in the past, done quite well in stone lifting, steel bending, grip strength, powerlifting, and bodybuilding (at least to my own satisfaction, and considering that I have always been a natural athlete). But I have not done all at the same time. I have focused on one area until I reached a certain benchmark, and have then gone on to something else. I was always aware that my strength in some area(s) might decrease when I change my focus, but the trick is to be fine with that.

You can, and should, make sure that you have a basic routine that trains all of the basic movement patterns, to have some balance and maintain your full-body strength. However, you should not expect to get better at every area at the same time. It is absolutely fine to let some areas *rest* completely for some time, and to only *maintain* your strength in others. If you do make progress in areas that are not your focus, by chance, all the better! But do not expect it and do not try to force it.

Also, remember that there are many ways to train the individual movement patterns. Do not dogmatically include exercises, just because you are used to them or because somebody tells you to. Some exercises can take a lot of energy away from your focus. If necessary, do without squats – the sacred cow of modern trainees – for half a year. There is no law in the world that can force you to do squats.

The same is true for the bench press. If you decide that you want to become better at your military shoulder press, focus on this exercise and leave the bench press away for a couple of months (or minimize your bench press training). There is nothing wrong with this. You will have more energy to improve your shoulder press, because you waste less energy on the bench press.

I will now provide an example of how this can be put into practice. Let us assume you want to become like an oldtime strongman and have, for the moment, decided to learn three different types of classic feats of strength: nail bending, card tearing, and a one arm push press. Nail bending, whether you do it with the underhand or overhand technique, is a feat that requires mostly great strength from the forearms. Card tearing is a grip strength feat. In the one arm push press the weak link is explosive shoulder strength. Keeping this in mind, you also want to maintain your current overall body strength. You have only limited time available, because you have a regular job and a partner, and decide that three workouts per week are sufficient. This will make sure you get plenty of rest, to then enter your workouts with full energy. Based on these assumptions, you could change the routine above to the following:

Monday (walking, running, jumping/dexterity 1):
- ◆ Squats
- ◆ Leg curl
- ◆ Sledgehammer levering
- ◆ Nail bending

Tuesday:
- ◆ Rest day

Wednesday (throwing):
- ◆ Barbell push press
- ◆ One-arm push press
- ◆ Kettlebell swings

Thursday:
- ◆ Rest day

Friday (lifting/dexterity 2/climbing):
- ◆ Deadlifts
- ◆ Thick bar deadlifts
- ◆ Pinch lift
- ◆ Hand gripper training
- ◆ Card tearing
- ◆ Pull ups

Saturday (swimming and dancing):
- ♦ Swimming in the morning
- ♦ Dancing in the evening with spouse

Sunday:
- ♦ Rest day

This is still a large undertaking, but, in contrast to the routine I presented earlier, it is at least manageable. First of all, I did away with the bench press, so that you can really focus on overhead lifting for now. I clearly separated your nail bending and card tearing days, because both put a lot of stress on the hands. To do this, I had to pair the nail bending day with your leg training, which is an arbitrary choice. But you could bend your nails in between your squat sets, for example, to make sure you have ample energy for these, and do not approach them after all your heavy squatting, when your energy is gone. Friday focuses on grip strength exercises, in particular *three different types* of grip strength training: thick bar lifting, pinch grip exercises, and hand gripper training. All of these will help you with card tearing. (By the way, how do you make progress in card tearing? Quite simply, you start with few cards and every once in a while you increase the amount of cards you tear in one go.) On Mondays and Wednesdays you have rather few different exercises per workout, but this does not hurt. You can do more sets per exercise, for example, or simply have more intense, but shorter workouts, which saves you time. You have four rest days per week, the evenings of which you can spend with nutritious meals and your partner, to work on your relationship and life quality while you let your muscles grow. The movement pattern of *hitting* is not in the plan, but you might want to train it with a few sit-ups in the mornings, or in between your other exercises, or at the end of each workout. The same is true of *biting*. You can train the neck muscles involved in this movement pattern with a few rubber band exercises every now and then. In sum, this workout plan is ambitious, but still minimalistic and simplistic. It puts a clear focus on a limited number of goals.

11. How to change your focus over time

Now that I have explained why it is important to focus on a limited number of goals, i.e. feats of strength, at the same time, I want to talk a little bit about how one can nevertheless become a versatile all-round oldtime strongman by changing his focus ever so often. Of course, there are endless possibilities of doing this, and people had success with very different approaches in this respect. However, there are some interesting aspects to consider and some recommendations I want to make.

First of all, it is advisable to have built a solid foundation of overall body strength before even going into specialized training for feats of strength. Anyone who has already some years of experience lifting weights, with basic exercises like the squat, deadlift, bench press, shoulder press, and barbell rows – all done with heavy loads and in a medium-to-low repetition range, like five to ten repetitions per set – is better qualified for oldtime strongman training than a regular person from the street who has never touched a weight in his life. There are exceptions to this, for example if someone has a history of hard physical labour over several years. This is an equally good, if not better, prerequisite.

If one also plans to perform feats of strength in front of an audience one day, it could also not hurt to have gained a certain amount of muscle mass already. People will buy into the claim that someone *is* strong, much faster when the person also *looks* strong. If the athlete has performed the exercises above also in the medium repetition range for some years – say eight to ten repetitions per set – and also regularly performed minor exercises like biceps curls, triceps extensions, and wrist curls, this should have been taken care of as well.

As a side note, I should add once more that the assumption that one must *look* strong to be a successful performing oldtime strongman, is one that has been disproved plenty of times in the past. I personally know several oldtime strongmen who have incredible strength, and perform mind-blowing feats of strength, although they are only averagely built. This can have the effect of *amplifying* the awe their performance inspires in an audience, because their otherworldly strength comes as even more of a surprise. Arthur Saxon has commented on this as well, saying, as early as 1906: "It is quite wrong to endeavour to fix a man's ability by his measurements, also to gauge a man's strength from muscular photos" (Saxon 36).

In any case, the next aspect to consider is how some feats of strength complement others. I should say that grip strength, for example, is a prerequisite for many different feats of strength. Most lifting and bending feats benefit from a strong grip, besides the fact that many of the classic feats of strength are grip strength feats in themselves. Therefore, it might be a good idea to see grip strength training and grip strength feats as a next step after a basic full-body training as described above. Once one has mastered all sorts of grip strength feats, he will have an easier time with lifting and bending feats.

Another aspect to consider is age. There is no denying the fact that everyone is an involuntary victim of the wheels of time. There is no escaping the ageing of your body. This being said, some strength feats and exercises are indeed more suitable for young trainees. However, other strength exercises can be performed – and some types of strength maintained – up to a very high age.

First of all, consider that there are three basic types of strength: explosive strength, maximum strength, and strength endurance. These types of strength "age" in that order: *Explosive strength* athletes perform best at a relatively young age, say, until their mid-twenties. *Maximum strength* can be built and increased up until middle age, at least until someone is 40 years of age – although I have seen many people dramatically increase their maximum strength beyond the age of 40. *Strength endurance* (which is the least relevant to an oldtime strongman) can be built and increased up until a high age. Even people in their fifties and sixties can display fantastic strength endurance. By the same logic, these types of strength can be maintained for a shorter or longer period of time, with explosive strength being the hardest to maintain up until a high age. Most classic oldtime strongman feats are maximum strength feats, but there are also explosive strength feats, like the push press, or any throwing feats, like the shot put, or some of the Highland Games disciplines. Thus, to be very straight and honest, if you want to excel in explosive strength feats, you would be well advised to focus on these at the start of your career, when you are still young (younger than twenty or in your early twenties).

With regard to maximum strength feats, there is obviously a wide range of feats. As a general rule, the more basic the exercise is, i.e. the more large muscle groups are involved, the less well the exercise ages – especially when the exercise mobilizes a muscle chain than crosses the mid-section of your body. The standing overhead press, the squat, the deadlift, stone lifting, and so on, put a lot of stress on your whole body, including lower back, hips, etc. As you age, and as your body begins to show tear and wear, it will become increasingly difficult to excel at these exercises. Maximum strength exercises with a more limited movement chain, or with a limited movement range (and therefore less prone to injuries), can theoretically be performed until a higher age. The bench press is one example. It is a rather comfortable exercise, done while lying on a cushioned bench. Also, consider the difference between the squat and a hip lift: While you lift much heavier weights in a hip lift than in a squat, a hip lift is performed across a very limited range of motion and much less dependent on intact knees, lower back, etc.

I should also add that some people would probably divide maximum strength into two different subcategories: 1) pure muscle strength, and 2) tendon and ligament strength. The common perception is that many of the classic feats of strength, like steel bending and grip strength feats, demand a greater proportion of what these people call tendon and ligament strength. Based on their observations, this type of strength is supposed to age better, and therefore such feats of strength are believed to be possible at a higher age compared to pure muscle strength exercises (which include most of the common weightlifting exercises). Also – so the theory goes – tendon and ligament strength is more dependent on the time factor to be built, i.e. it takes longer to be built, and it does not react so much to the abuse of substances (as pure muscle strength obviously does).

I have no scientific biological or sports science data to support these assumptions, but I believe that there is something to them. Exercises like grip strength and steel bending feats can be trained, excelled at, and performed, up to a higher age than the basic, common weightlifting exercises. This is good news to those who want to train oldtime strongman feats for many years to come, but bad news for aspiring stone lifters, for example, who have already reached a certain age. Natural stone lifting is not that different from deadlifting and related exercises. I thus consider it mostly a pure muscle strength feat, and advise you to start your training on it early, if you can. However, even with this theory under consideration, as tendon and ligament strength takes longer to develop than pure muscle strength, you should also not postpone the training for this type of strength for too long.

By the way, when I say that tendon and ligament strength can be maintained up to a relatively high age (and often with little training or no training at all, i.e. it is very durable), I do not want you to think that it does not cause tear and wear in your body. It should be obvious that extreme stress on the body – and this includes any kind of strength training – causes the kind of strain that can later in your life lead to very uncomfortable and troublesome issues – however great the benefit of strength training to your body may be, compared to no activity at all.

I have already mentioned several times the role that appearance plays for an oldtime strongman, and that I do not consider looks, or, more precisely, an overly muscular-looking body, a necessity for an oldtime strongman. I also said that an average-looking body can sometimes have the effect of making the displayed strength of a person appear like a cosmic phenomenon or something of the sort, and therefore all the more impressive (as a side note, I have also seen the opposite phenomenon – a so-called strongman who looked big and powerful, but whose feats of strength were only magical illusions. You can imagine that I am not overly fond of this).

Nevertheless, I fully understand if you have the ambition to *look* as strong as you *are*. If you plan to perform on stage, it can also benefit your show if your visual appearance already commands respect before you even do anything. Thus, if you want to train for looks – which I will now call bodybuilding training for the sake of simplicity – be advised that this kind of training consists in essence of sets in a medium repetition range, between eight and twelve, but up to a maximum of 15 repetitions. This constitutes a comparatively light stress on the body and joints. Bodybuilding training can therefore be performed up to a much higher age than maximum strength training (not to mention explosive strength training).

In my opinion you should not really spend too much time on feats of endurance strength while you are young. You can consider them a last resort, once you have reached a high age and want to achieve new goals (which I would by all means encourage you to do).

Taking all of this into consideration, here is one possibility of how to structure your training and priorities over time, in a chronological order:

- ◆ Olympic weightlifting training in a respected weightlifting club (starting in early youth with mostly technique training, then continuing with serious competitive weightlifting, up to about your early twenties).
- ◆ Maintaining light weightlifting training and switching to oldtime strongman training, with a special focus on grip strength feats, and a second focus on steel bending feats (from early twenties to mid-forties).
- ◆ Switching from light weightlifting training to a considerate bodybuilding training of ten to 15 repetitions per set, with an aim of improving your looks. Doing oldtime strongman feats on a constant level, mostly to maintain tendon and ligament strength. Increasingly play gentle and safe endurance (strength) sports, like swimming and hiking.

This order will have several benefits: Olympic weightlifting training can be taken up quite early in a professional club, where people will take care that you learn the proper technique without ruining your young body, for example by using too heavy weights too early. Later on, as you add weight to the bar, you will learn universal, full-body exercises (clean, snatch, press, etc.) that will automatically build a versatile, strong, balanced, and even good-looking body (if you keep your body fat low).

Early enough, in your twenties, you start reducing the extreme stress on your joints that competitive Olympic weightlifting consists of, before you ruin your body. Instead, and early enough in time, you take up serious grip strength training, and eventually steel bending training, to build tendon and ligament strength over time. At the same time, you continue with a light weightlifting workout to maintain overall body strength.

At the right point in time, you stop being over-ambitious and stop risking injuries, by being happy with the level of strength you have reached so far, and only try to maintain it for as long as possible. Instead of your weightlifting exercises, which cause lots of stress on your joints even when exercised with lighter weights, you switch to a considerate bodybuilding training, enjoying how your looks improve (or, at least, do not deteriorate). Thus, your body will look better as you get older, which is the opposite of what people would expect. As paradoxical as it sounds, you will be able to delay the gradual and natural ageing of your physical appearance for a considerable amount of time. Increasing the percentage of endurance (strength) training as you get older will help you to be active up until a high age, and be great for your heart and circulatory system.

Here is another example:

♦ Starting with light bodybuilding training in your youth, including the basic full-body exercises with mediocre weights and in a relatively high repetition range.

♦ Switching to competitive powerlifting training in your late teens, increasing the weights on the powerlifting exercises and reducing the proportion of complementary bodybuilding exercises. Taking up natural stone lifting at the same time.

♦ Gradually taking up grip strength training.

♦ By the age of 30, switching to a serious and versatile oldtime strongman training, doing powerlifting exercises only occasionally to maintain overall body strength.

♦ Gradually reducing the weight in powerlifting exercises and increasing repetition-range, maintaining oldtime strongman feats, increasingly playing gentle and safe endurance (strength) sports, like swimming and hiking (see above).

This would be a way to go if you do not have the possibility to train in a weightlifting club. Bodybuilding and powerlifting training can practically be done in any commercial gym or in a home gym. Powerlifting training and stonelifting benefit from each other – the lifting strength and chest strength of your powerlifting training will help you lift huge stones. The same is true of grip strength training, which can be done on the side, without inhibiting your powerlifting training too much. The rest of this example is similar to the example above, although it leaves out the training for looks. Gradually switching to more endurance (strength) training as you reach a higher age is always the best way to go.

12. How to choose a gym, or make your own home gym. And what equipment you need.

Now that I have talked a little bit about *what* exercises an oldtime strongman can perform and *how* they can be combined over the course of a week, and altered over the years, let me turn to the question of *where* one can perform these workouts, i.e. what kind of location and equipment one needs for an efficient oldtime strongman training.

As with many aspects connected to oldtime strongman training, there are no rules or laws set in stone. Instead, there is a lot of room for creativity, which is part of the beauty of it. I have had exceptional training results in all kinds of environments, including a tiny cellar compartment with an earthen floor, with only about four cubic metres. However, there are certain prerequisites that, if your gym fulfils them, will give you an advantage and guarantee a more efficient training.

For example: since I believe that a country life is the best life for any person, I believe it is also the best environment for an oldtime strongman. There are always exceptions, of course. The famous oldtime strongman Joseph Greenstein (1893-1977), also known as "The Mighty Atom", lived and trained in New York City and honed his legendary strength in an urban environment. However, ideally, an oldtime strongman has a house with a large garden, a roofed home gym (which can be outdoors), and a small workshop to build and maintain his own equipment and props. This constellation is preferable to any commercial gym, because – depending of the feats the trainee wants to train for – oldtime strongman training will require a lot of room to move, a ground that can take damage, and the possibility to use homemade equipment. If you are alone during your workouts, you can train for uncommon feats of strength you are not very good at yet, without the fear of making a fool of yourself – as you would in a much-frequented gym.

However, if you do not live together with someone who shares your interests, the downside is that you have no assistant, whom you might need for other feats of strength – no human weights or spotters, for example. So in the ideal case, you have both: a home gym with avid room to experiment, and some kind of gym where you meet like-minded people who motivate you or help you out if you need assistance.

As oldtime strongman training is a little known sport, it is unlikely that you will find many companions who want to train in the exact same disciplines as you. But you might at least find a near weightlifting or powerlifting gym with all the basic equipment, like heavy barbells, dumbbells, racks, and a lifting floor where it is no problem if you drop these weights. Here you can perform some of the basic exercises to complement your specialized training: squats, bench press, overhead lifts, etc. Here you can establish relationships with strong people who will have some understanding if you ask them to come over to your place at the weekend, because you need some volunteers for a back lift of 18 grown men.

Now, let us assume you have the opportunity to live in the country and set up your own home gym. What kind of equipment will you need? Of course, it depends on the feats you want to train for, but let us assume you want to become a kind of universalist. Then, the following equipment and tools will enable a multifaceted oldtime strongman training:

- Lots of weight plates, with varying steps of progression, like 20kg (44lbs), 10kg (22lbs), 5kg (11lbs), 2.5kg (5.5lbs), and 1.25kg (2.75lbs)
- At least one weightlifting bar and two shorter bars to make barbells and dumbbells of varying weight
- A loading pin, i.e. a vertical bar with a hook on top that you can load with weight plates
- Sand bags are convenient sometimes
- One or two natural lifting stones, for example a lighter and a heavier one
- A few kettlebells, or at least one
- A vice
- Lots of leftover pieces of leather in varying thickness and quality
- Some cloths
- A calliper
- Some chains and shackles and/or pieces of rope, e.g. for improvised lifting or towing feats
- Chalk
- A floor or ground that is resistant to dropping weights
- Tape for your fingers, to keep training when your skin in torn
- A sledgehammer
- A power rack
- A bench
- A sturdy box for leftover, bent steel, to take to the local scrap dealer once a year
- A bookshelf with some reference books
- Pen and paper

With these pieces of equipment you will be able to train your overall strength with all the basic exercises, and to try all sorts of oldtime strongman feats – improvising and experimenting along the way. *Weights* and *bars* are self-explanatory. You will need them for any basic weightlifting exercise and for any other lifting feat you want to try. For the latter, a *loading pin* is the most comfortable way to attach weight, for example if you want to try teeth lifts or one-finger lifts. On the other hand, if you want to train more advances feats, like balancing feats, or feats with human weights, you might want to use *sand bags* as weights, as they cause less damage to your floor (and you) if they drop. By the way, sandbag training is a great way to train overall strength as well. *Lifting stones* are obviously for natural stone lifting, but they can also serve as additional weight for feats where you need all the weight you can get, like a back or harness lift. Also, they are for free and can be disposed easily, without regret. *Kettlebells* are quite old school (if you find some that are made of metal) and kettlebell juggling is a wonderful oldtime strongman pastime.

A *vice* is helpful for lots of bending feats. As mentioned above, coins, nails, horseshoes, wrenches etc. can be bent with the teeth when clamped in a vice. Also, a vice is necessary if you want to cut steel bars, nails, etc. to fit your needs. *Leather* and *cloths* you will need to experiment with steel bending feats. Be it nails, horseshoes, or steel bars, you will need different padding for different feats, and you will need to experiment with varying sizes, thickness, etc. A *calliper* is an underestimated tool for an oldtime strongman, as it is needed to measure the thickness of steel bars, etc. for comparison and progression. *Chalk* is almost indispensable for grip strength training and record attempts. *Chains with shackles* and/or *ropes* will help with any experimenting with common and exotic feats of strength. Of course, I mean strong, welded chains. But you can also collect some chains for chain breaking feats. Preferably, you then look out for such chains where the links are simply bent and not welded, as it is very hard to break any welded chain (but not impossible, if it is a relatively small chain).

The sturdy *floor or ground* might seem obvious, but it is not something to be taken lightly. Training in the upper floor of a regular house, for example, is irresponsible for an oldtime strongman. Also, training while having to worry about dropping weights is disturbing. *Tape* has helped me on many occasions when my skin was torn, or about to tear, and goes a long way to make sure you can keep up your training. The kind of tape that rock climbers use works very well (For the sake of hygiene and health, it might also not hurt to have a first-aid-kit ready, and some strong alcohol – not to drink, but to disinfect small wounds. However, if you have any larger, serious injuries, please go see a doctor. If not taken care of, they can seriously inhibit your oldtime strongman career. The sad fate of "*Eisenkönig*" Sigmund Breitbart shall serve as a warning here).

A *sledgehammer* is a wonderful tool for an oldtime strongman. It can be used for levering exercises to strengthen your forearms, which can be turned into a feat of strength itself (Slim "The Hammer-Man", a protégé of "The Mighty Atom" Joseph Greenstein, built a whole strongman career on this one feat of strength). Beyond this, a sledgehammer can be used for finger walking, an additional exercise to strengthen your fingers, which I talk about in my book *Grip Strength*. Also, if you care to get hold of a large loader tyre, you will obviously need a sledgehammer to perform the (very effective) hitting exercises I talked about above. I should also mention my colleague Mighty Mike from Canada, who performs a juggling feat with a sledgehammer. I have seen these feats live and the reactions of the audience were wonderful.

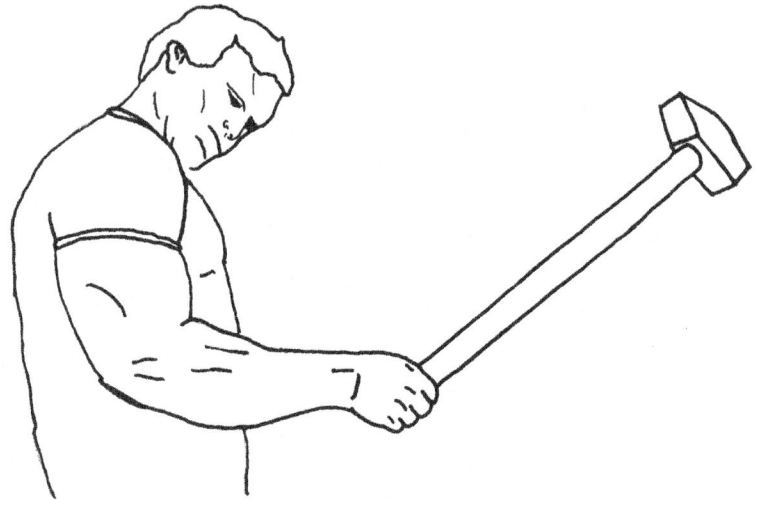

Figure 12.1 Levering exercise with a sledgehammer.

If you do some research on the golden age of the strongmen, you will realize that the *power rack*, as it is commonly called, is a relatively recent invention, despite its apparent simplicity. This is so because a rack is mostly necessary and used for variations of the bench press and the back squat – two exercises that require safety measures when performed with heavy weights. However, these two exercises were rather uncommon in the days of the oldtime strongmen. Overhead presses predominated, and for overhead lifting a power rack is not necessary. Even if you train alone, you can simply drop the barbell to the floor.

As a side note, you might actually want to consider training according to this spirit – performing a true oldtime weightlifting training and disregarding the back squat and bench press altogether. You will still be able to build a strong and balanced body. Although I still perform both the back squat and the bench press myself, I believe that an overdeveloped chest from excessive bench pressing leads to a rather disproportionate body.

Claiming that a strongman can do without the back squat, will probably cause an outcry among modern trainees. The back squat has, in recent years, garnered the reputation of an absolute must, and an exercise that separates men from boys, so to say. This is, of course, only proof of how beginners tend to repeat what they hear or read elsewhere, without any reflection or real knowledge of the subject. An Olympic weightlifter, for example, will build tremendous strength and a very well balanced and proportionate body, without ever performing the bench press or the back squat, if he wants to. Also, you will make your life easier, because you save the money and space needed for such a cumbersome contraption as a power rack.

But I digress. If, despite these thoughts, you do decide to include the bench press and the back squat in your training regimen, the easiest and safest way to do so at home is with a power rack. Then, on the positive side, a power rack will also allow you to experiment with such exciting endeavours as partial deadlifts or partial overhead presses, so-called lockouts. I have always been particularly fond of such and have, for example, lifted up to 450kg (993lbs) in partial deadlifts (with lifting straps). This in itself is no feat of strength, but I believe it has helped me with other exercises and feats, like stone lifting and the harness lift – let alone regular deadlifts.

Talking about the bench press, this exercise is the main reason why you should have a *bench* in your home gym, so if you decide to delete the bench press from your workout plan, you will not be in so much need of a bench. However, a bench may come in handy for lots of other exercises, like seated wrist curls, or simply to rest in between sets.

A *box* to collect the scrap metal you have bent is a nice motivation, as it demonstrates all the work you have done in terms of steel bending over the year. Also, if you collect all your bent metal in this one place, you will always know where it all is when you want to take it to the local scrap dealer once a year. This, by the way, will not make you rich, as the price for scrap metal is very low and can mostly be disregarded. However, it is a nice ritual and the only right thing you can do with all this bent metal: recycle it, so that it can be turned into something useful again. The only other alternative is to keep it in your home as a trophy or keepsake, but I do this only with very meaningful objects.

A *bookshelf with some reference books* is not really necessary in a home gym, as you can keep all your books on strength training in your living room or personal library as well. However, a bookshelf in your gym can create a nice and cosy ambience, in contrast to the cold and sterile atmosphere that some of the places usually used for home gyms radiate (like cellars or garages).

As a side note, I generally regret the design of modern training locations, most of which are not very cosy and inviting at all. The furniture and equipment of these is mostly of artificial material and badly designed. Compare this to some of the photographs of the gyms and weightlifting rooms of 120 years ago: You will realize the exclusive use of natural, and visually pleasing building material, like walnut wood and brass, and a sophisticated and aesthetically pleasing interior design, nothing short of some *Gründerzeit* inner-city palais. But I digress again. *Pen and paper* are indispensable tools to track progression. I will talk about this below.

While all of the items above are helpful in a home gym, do not make the mistake to run out and purchase everything before you start with your training. An oldtime strongman gym is not built overnight. Equipment must be of high quality and durable, and acquired piece by piece. Also, opportunities will come up where you can get hold of the one or the other used item for little money, or for free. Start with some basics, keep your eyes open, invest in a good piece of equipment now and then, and give your oldtime strongman home gym time to grow. It is like a quality home workshop.

Once you have a basic home gym, or at least all the equipment you believe you need to work on your first specific goal, I would suggest you also keep your eyes open for some of the following pieces and consumables. If you have enough patience, you will probably be able to collect them in considerable quantities without any cost. They are required for various feats of strength. Even if you are not interested in learning and performing any of these at the moment, at some point in time you might at least want to try them. Who knows, maybe you will change your mind later on to focus on the one or the other indeed.

- Metal pipes (can be used for thick bar training)
- Frying pans
- Used horseshoes
- Steel bars and construction steel
- Spikes and nails
- Phone books
- Decks of cards
- Hot water bottles

I think most of these objects are self-explanatory, and it is obvious for which feats of strength they serve. *Metal pipes* with various diameters and lengths can be used for many different kinds of thick bar training to strengthen your grip. If you find a very short metal pipe, you can build some kind of handle for one-hand thick bar lifts. If you find a medium-length pipe, you can repurpose it as a thick bar dumbbell. If you find a long enough pipe with the proper diameter, this will be the cheapest thick handled barbell available.

Frying pans make for a feat of strength that is quite popular with audiences (rolling up a frying pan), but actually I am not very fond of it. The reasons being: 1) There are huge differences between the qualities of different brands of pans, making this feat anything from extremely difficult to extremely easy. Any type of record with this feat, like someone having rolled up so-and-so many frying pans within such-and-such a time, is very relative and can either be an impressive performance, or not very difficult at all – nobody can tell who has not looked at the pans. 2) This feat is only possible with modern, coated pans, which are not very visually pleasing, and often consist of artificial material to a large part, which is hard to be recycled. Thus, the feat creates a lot of unnecessary waste. However, if someone offers you an old frying pan that is waste already, i.e. the person was about to dispose it either way (which, I regret to say, happens frequently in our modern throw-away society), then why not accept the offer and use the pan to attempt a feat of strength?

Decks of cards, steel bars, spikes, and *phone books* are obvious. These you can collect to try feats like card-tearing, steel and nail bending, and phone book tearing. They create only little, easily recyclable waste. As a side note, phone book tearing is a feat I am also not too fond of, because there are techniques to do this that practically amount to cheating. From watching, the amateur cannot tell the difference. Also, phone books have practically disappeared in recent years, and there are some children nowadays who do not even know what a phone book is. This makes the feat a bit odd, but perhaps it will be considered nostalgic in a few more years to come. The question will then be where to get the phone books from.

Used horseshoes are the cheapest way to start practising the art of horseshoe bending, as I explained earlier. By starting out with used horseshoes, which might be bent easily if well worn in the centre part, you can experiment with the technique without having to spend money on new, unused horseshoes. A riding stable will usually give away used horseshoes for free.

The feat of blowing up a *hot water bottle* until it bursts is as dangerous as impressive. My good colleague Georges Christen from Luxembourg is the world champion in this feat. There are, of course, differences in quality in hot water bottles as well. However, I should say that blowing up a hot water bottle of even mediocre quality, until it bursts, requires tremendously strong lungs and great courage. Look out for opportunities to get old, used water bottles if you ever plan to gather up the courage to give this feat a serious try.

Now that I have talked about some of the *material* items an oldtime strongman might need, let me add a few words on a very different kind of resource. An oldtime strongman also needs some kind of network of *people*. Remember that the times of the true oldtime strongmen were very different to ours. It was a world of much more face-to-face communication and interpersonal interaction. A strongman of the old days would live and strive in some small village with a local weightlifting club, where he is in good contact with the blacksmith around the corner, a farmer with a couple of oxen in his stables, and the local craftsmen whom he would meet in the pub in the evening. There, he would ask them over a beer if they had time on Sunday afternoon to help with an attempt in the "human link" feat, where the strongman holds back two or four horses with two arm slings. He would ask the local brewer whether he could spare four of his carriage horses for an hour, and the saddler whether he could bring some sturdy straps to use as slings. Of course they would agree, because they would welcome change in their everyday lives, and have no other plans for Sunday. Also, they would gladly provide the desired items, and the whole village would watch and cheer the attempt of the strongman.

In our modern times, especially in urban environments, things are very different. People do not know you personally, are too busy, or are simply not interested in your business. They are already overloaded with impressions, incoming messages, and diversions, throughout the whole day.

However, this does not mean that you should not at least make an attempt to recreate the atmosphere of the old days. Build a network of people around you, and connect with local scrap metal dealers, horse smiths, blacksmiths, carpenters, shoemakers, doctors, lawyers, and sensible local strength enthusiasts. Establish personal, life-long relationships with people you might need to supply steel for bending, to build equipment for you, to consult in case of injury or legal questions, and companions who support you with encouragement, friendly competition, and help. Build a foundation of trust, be a faithful customer, do not just chase after the cheapest price, and buy locally, or do not order your equipment without ever personally meeting your suppliers if you can avoid it. Your trusted dealers will know you, your needs, and what you are up to, and they will soon get to know you as a nostalgic idealist and dreamer, and ask no more questions. Invest in real-life relationships in the same way as you invest in your equipment.

Talking about investing in equipment: Let me emphasize again that all of your equipment can be old, second hand, used, and rusty. All of this does not matter. On the contrary, the more worn your equipment is, the more "oldtime" it will feel. This will help you to mentally connect with the golden age of the strongmen, and enter the mind-set of past, simpler, and harder times.

The good thing about oldtime strongman training is that most of the equipment needed does practically not age. I own weight plates I purchased over 20 years ago, for my first workouts, and they work as well as they did back then. They have only become a bit rusty, and even this I could have avoided if had taken better care, i.e. stored them properly, and oiled them now and then.

An oldtime strongman should not give in to the temptations of the modern world of consumerism. He should act wisely, be considerate, and think sustainably. He should ignore the announcement of new, revolutionary pieces of equipment, and avoid spontaneous, intuitive purchases. In these days, it seems relatively easy to sell so-called "revolutionary" training equipment that, in truth, has just not passed the test of time yet. Still, it attracts buyers with unrealistic promises of strength and fitness gains yet unheard of. Many of these pieces of equipment lack durability and quality. Therefore, one should plan each purchase carefully, and let a buying decision settle for some time, to give oneself the opportunity to ponder whether the purchase is really necessary. Invest in few and basic, but quality pieces of equipment, bit by bit, with the mind-set that you will keep them for the rest of your life. Also, an oldtime strongman should avoid *conspicuous consumption,* i.e. buying items that are meant to impress other people.

In sum, when you plan to purchase a piece of equipment, always consider the following aspects first:

- ◆ Necessity: Is the piece of equipment *really* necessary for me to reach my strength goals?
- ◆ Urgency: Is the piece of equipment really necessary *now* for me to reach my strength goals?
- ◆ Durability: Is the quality of the product such that it will last for a long time? Will it outlive my strongman career? Will it outlive me?
- ◆ Space: Considering that I will keep the equipment for such a long time, do I really have the space to store it? Will it be a burden when I move to a new place? Will it be a burden to the people living with me, my spouse, children, etc., as it will take up space they might need?

- ◆ Alternatives: If it is a new piece of equipment, is there a used, second hand alternative? Or could I, perhaps, build an equivalent piece of equipment myself? What are my options to save money here?
- ◆ Intrinsic value: How much of its value will the piece of equipment retain once I have used it for some time? Will I have the option to sell it later on without losing too much money?

As an oldtime strongman, you have to get rid of the mind-set that you constantly have to buy new training equipment. You are not running a commercial gym and do not have to own lots of new, shiny machines to make the impression that your business is running well.

The same is true for your gym clothes. The most important factors here are that they are comfortable, give you ample space to move, are durable, and protect you from natural influences, for example, cold weather. Oldtime strongman training can mean a lot of tear and wear to your clothes – consider stone lifting, for example – so do not make fashion or outward appearance a priority. If you ever plan to become a performing oldtime strongman and do shows for money, or if you even want to live off your performances one day, you will have to learn to be thrifty any way, as this kind of lifestyle involves great financial risks. Then, of course, you should also remember that your outward appearance does *very well matter* if you step in front of an audience! But more on this later.

If you want to know where I train, and with what kind of equipment, I will shortly explain it here. I own quite a lot of equipment I have collected over the years. Sometimes I feel it is more than I would like to own. More than once I asked myself where to store it all. I have several long and short bars and lots of weight plates with a 30mm (1.2in) diameter hole, some of them more than 20 years old. My first 10kg (22lbs) dumbbell set I got as a birthday present when I was nine. Since then, I continuously expanded my home gym, and bought more weights myself, or received them as birthday and Christmas presents. I remember well when I was a teenager, and my mother gave me two 20kg (44lbs) weight plates for Christmas. She had carried them all the way from the bus stop to our house in the Tyrolean village where I grew up, through streets covered with thick layers of snow.

I still own most of these weights, and a very cheap and wobbly bench I bought from my pocket money when I was 14. It is meant for a maximum load of 100kg (221lbs), although, by the time I was 17, I bench pressed 160kg (353lbs) on it. Sadly, I lost two of my 20kg (44lbs) weight plates later on, as I had left them lying in the garden of a house where I lived as a student. The guy living on the second floor was an ex-convict, who, when he moved out, took all moveable items in the furnished apartment with him, plus two of my weight plates.

I also own two Olympic weightlifting bars, lots of weight plates with a 50mm (2in) hole, a very sturdy power rack, a proper bench, three kettlebells (One of these is an antiquity I received as a present from a Thuringian fan, and at least 70 years old. In terms of quality, it is the best I ever saw), several hand grippers, an anvil, a lifting keg filled with sand, a lifting stone, an Atlas stone, a sledgehammer, a Rolling Thunder deadlift handle, a Hub lift, some home-made pieces of equipment, and, of course, all my props for my shows, including consumables like nails, horseshoes, decks of cards, and so on. I have two large wooden boxes, in one of which I store items like frying pans, phone books, spikes, chains, shackles, etc. I come across, in case I might need them. In the other box I store bent nails, horseshoes, and steel bars, until I discard them once per year, as described above.

I have four locations where I can train, all of which cost me very little or no money. 1) I can train at home, in my basement, where I can do all basic exercises in a space of roughly four cubic metres. It is a very dusty and dirty place, the cellar of an old *Gründerzeit* city house with an earthen floor. 2) I can train on the open air site of a circus, where I do anything I have to do, or want to do, outdoors, like stone lifting and carrying. 3) There is a local powerlifting gym where I can train, which has a nice atmosphere, as it is rather small, cramped, and dirty. It also has all of the necessary equipment for serious powerlifting training, including my own power rack, bench, and Olympic weights. I gave these to the gym as a permanent loan, so that other people can use them as well. 4) I can also train at the gym of a municipal government not far away, reserved for local sports clubs. It has a very friendly atmosphere, a bit more space, and some roomy machines like leg presses etc. Still, it does not have the feel of a commercial gym.

All of these possibilities did not come out of nowhere, of course. It was partly by chance, and partly by being permanently on the lookout for opportunities, that I ended up with these different locations I can use for very little money – for which I am very grateful, by the way.

To sum up, oldtime strongman training is a very variable endeavour. How, where, and with what equipment one will train, depends very much on the chosen feats of strength, on personal preferences, on possibilities, and on the individual character of the trainee. In any case, an aspiring oldtime strongman has to think outside the box, as they say. He has to be creative and flexible with training equipment and location, to make sure he has the possibility to work on the feats of strength he wants to achieve.

This being said, I have made the experience that progress can be made in the most different locations and under many different circumstances. It is a fallacy to think that one is dependent on a certain place, equipment, training partners, atmosphere, time of day, or music, to train efficiently. It is often only a question of habit and being used to such circumstances. If one is forced to train in a very different environment from one day to another, his performance will certainly suffer momentarily. The trainee will then conclude that he *needs* his familiar atmosphere by all means. But this is not the case. As a rule of thumb, it takes about two weeks to become used to new surroundings. Then, one will be back on his prior level and make progress again from there. Thus, once habituated, one can literally train *anywhere*.

13. The appearance of an oldtime strongman: Body types and training for looks

Many will consider a section on *training for looks*, i.e. bodybuilding, a contradiction in a book on oldtime strongman training. They will consider it one of the assets of oldtime strength to be largely independent of looks, muscle mass, and body fat percentage. Let us recall the quote by Arthur Saxon from 1906: "It is quite wrong to endeavour to fix a man's ability by his measurements, also to gauge a man's strength from muscular photos" (Saxon 36). I completely agree with this quote. It has lost nothing of its relevance. Nevertheless, not all strongmen of the golden age looked at it from this perspective. Many considered it part of their performance, act, and marketing, to pose, flex their muscles, and to also *look* strong. As I explained above, I am also of the opinion that it can benefit a *performing* oldtime strongman to have visually impressive muscularity. Thus, I want to dedicate a few lines to the relation between oldtime *strength* and *looks* in terms of a muscular-looking body.

First of all – and this is where body types come into play – I should mention two important aspects: 1) The strongmen of the golden age came in all shapes and sizes, and there is no definite *look* of *the* oldtime strongman – quite the opposite: there was a great diversity. 2) It can lead to a lot of frustration, waste of time, and waste of energy, to try to force oneself to build a body that contradicts one's natural disposition and genetic potential.

Let me now have a closer look at aspect no. 1). In popular culture, and in the collective subconscious of our society, there exist various images of the oldtime strongman. One example would be a bald, chubby, not overly tall fellow with a red and white striped bathing suit, a black leather belt, and a black handlebar moustache, lifting a globe barbell. Any similar caricature will immediately make clear to a wide audience immediately what figure is being portrayed here – whether in a comic strip, in a film, or in a carnival costume – even if they cannot label it, because they are not familiar with the term "oldtime strongman" (which is any way only an arbitrary label for what was simply a "strong man" up until the end of World War II). But, when you look at actual photographs of historical strongmen of the golden age period, you will first of all realize that this prototype did never exist (I know of no single historical strongman who performed in a striped suit), and secondly – leaving the costume aside for a moment – that these strongmen were individuals with very individual body types and looks.

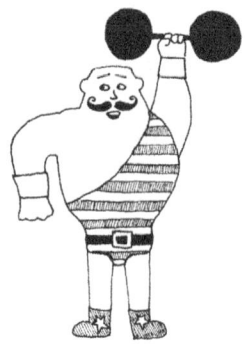

Figure 13.1 A stereotypical illustration of an oldtime strongman.

In the following, I want to undertake a broad categorization of these body types (I hope the reader will keep in mind that this is an arbitrary categorization that does not take into account that transitions were fluent). I suggest that there are four major oldtime strongman body types:

1. The wiry type
2. The brawny type
3. The overweight type
4. The giant

I would also argue that these different body types have, in one way or the other, and each to a smaller or larger degree, entered the collective subconscious as "strong men". But let me not spend too many thoughts on this any more and let me now take a closer look at the different types.

1. The wiry type: This is actually my favourite strongman type, because he has the element of surprise on his side. When wearing a shirt and jacket, he looks like a regular fellow from the street – except, perhaps, for his angular face, veiny forearms, thick wrists, and calloused hands. But when he takes his shirt off, his sinewy muscles, though not rounded and overdeveloped, but with deep cuts and covered with little fat, speak of a seasoned and experienced athlete who can "outgrip" and "outbend" any man from the street. These athletes, often not particularly tall either, provide living proof of the saying "size does not matter" (with regard to muscle size and height). Their assets are mostly feats of ligament strength, although a wiry athlete can also be a great deadlifter, for example. Typical

representatives of this type were Joseph "The Mighty Atom" Greenstein, or Adrian Peter Schmidt (1872-1944).

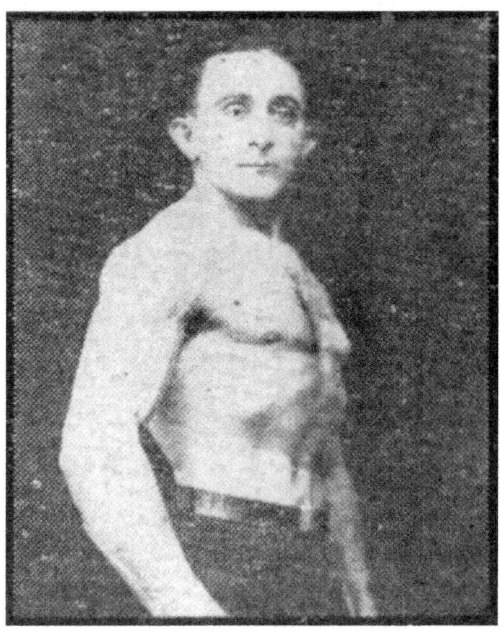

Figure 13.2 The wiry type: Joseph "The Mighty Atom" Greenstein.

2. The brawny type: These strongmen are probably the most versatile athletes: big and strong, with considerable muscle mass, and, if not literally "shredded" (they do not care enough about looks to go on a diet), without layers of fat that cover their muscles. Of course, an oldtime strongman does not have the kind of exaggerated, overblown, and bizarre muscle mass of a modern bodybuilder, but a dense, potent muscle mass that can do what it promises: broad shoulders, thick joints, huge thighs, round biceps, massive forearms, and a thick, brawny, and muscular waist. These men *look* strong (with clothes or without) and *are* strong. Typical brawny strongmen were Hermann Görner, Alexander Zass (188-1962), and, most prominently, George Hackenschmidt (1878-1968).

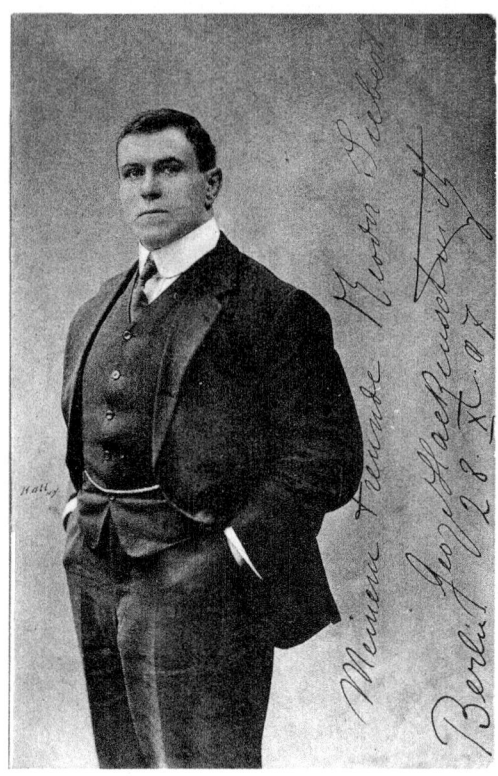

Figure 13.3 The brawny type: George Hackenschmidt.

3. The overweight type: This type is interesting, because it plays an important role in the concept of the "oldtime strongman" in the modern day collective subconscious. How often does it happen that an actor gets away with being cast as an oldtime strongman in a film, simply because he is tall, fat, and has a huge belly? For many people today, body mass equals strength. There is a small truth in this, as body mass can be utilized through inertia and as a counterweight for specific feats of strength. For example, all talented natural stonelifters have great body mass and height. There is only one downsize to this body type: an excessive body fat percentage carries several health risks. Nevertheless, some of the greatest strongmen of all times carried an amount of body fat that covered their considerable muscle mass, like Louis Cyr (1863-1912) or Karl Mörke (1889-1946). The epitome of the overweight oldtime strongman is probably Emil Naucke (1855-1900).

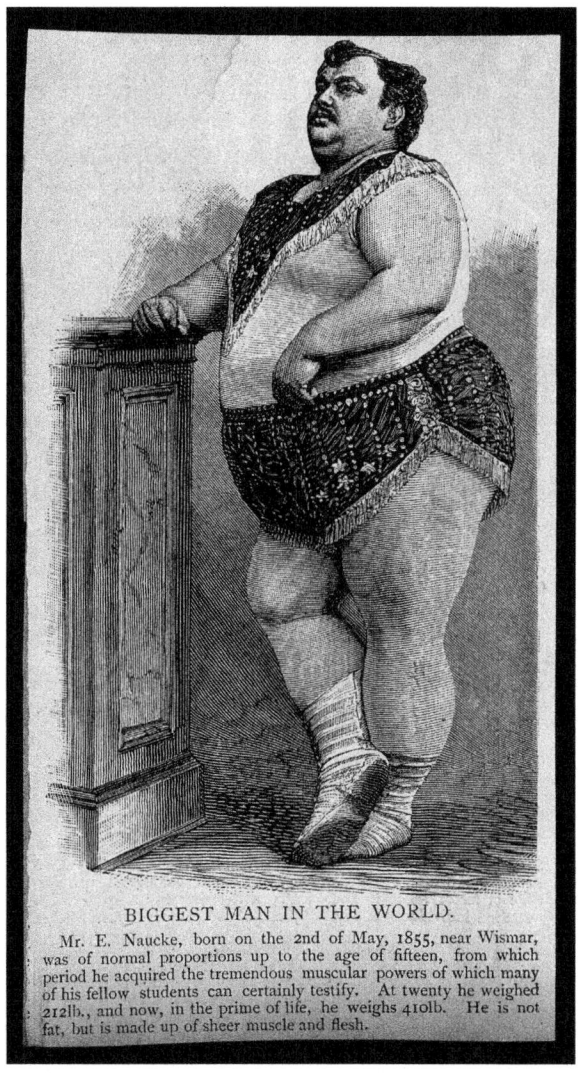

BIGGEST MAN IN THE WORLD.

Mr. E. Naucke, born on the 2nd of May, 1855, near Wismar, was of normal proportions up to the age of fifteen, from which period he acquired the tremendous muscular powers of which many of his fellow students can certainly testify. At twenty he weighed 212lb., and now, in the prime of life, he weighs 410lb. He is not fat, but is made up of sheer muscle and flesh.

Figure 13.4 The overweight type: Emil Naucke.

4. The giant: This type is related to the overweight type. In the popular perception, someone with a height above average, and a generally exaggerated body size, is automatically seen as strong and potent – even if this is so due to a medical condition. These men, for example if they suffer from acromegaly or gigantism, have the advantage that they are considered strong above average without having to perform any training with weights (despite the many sad discomforts caused by their condition). The

idea behind this perception might be that they are not necessarily built *differently* from other humans, but only in *larger proportions,* much like the giants from fairly tales. Therefore, they are considered stronger and more potent by such a proportion, simply by default, and not by their own desire. This asset can be combined with the overweight aspect. Thus, if you are overly tall *and* heavy, one could let you stand on a stage and introduce you as the strongman, without anyone daring to doubt your potency.

However, the truth is that although there are differences with regard to how strong someone can become through his genetic potential only, without any specialized training, I believe that the athlete who follows a rigorous workout plan will always have the potential to become *stronger* than anyone who does *not* train for it. Therefore, most strongmen of the giant type actually do belong into the fields of fiction, fantasy, fairy tale, and showmanship. This being said, some of the modern strongmen could also be counted to the giant type, although they obviously *do* train with weights.

If my reader, as an aspiring oldtime strongman, *does* care about his outward appearance in terms of muscularity (which he by no means must), the question he should ask himself is: "Towards which of these body types do I naturally tend?" The reason being that it is very difficult to transform one's body in order to fit a type for which one does not have the *inclination.* I have observed that most trainees, when they follow their preferred standard training and nutrition routine, according to their motivation and recuperation ability, as well as to their natural appetite and preferred nutrition, will tend towards a specific body weight and body type. If they have the discipline and desire, they will manage to significantly move away from their "standard", but it will require a conscious effort, like dieting, additional (cardiovascular) exercise, or forced feeding. Once they relax again, train how they feel, and eat how they feel, their body composition will swing back to their natural inclination. Thus, it is questionable if an aspiring oldtime strongman should aim for a significant body transformation at all. It will require a great effort, and energy that might better be invested in a focus on becoming stronger. For example, it is questionable whether Louis Cyr would ever have lifted such an astonishing number of pounds, if he had worried about counting calories and dieting to develop visible abdominal muscles.

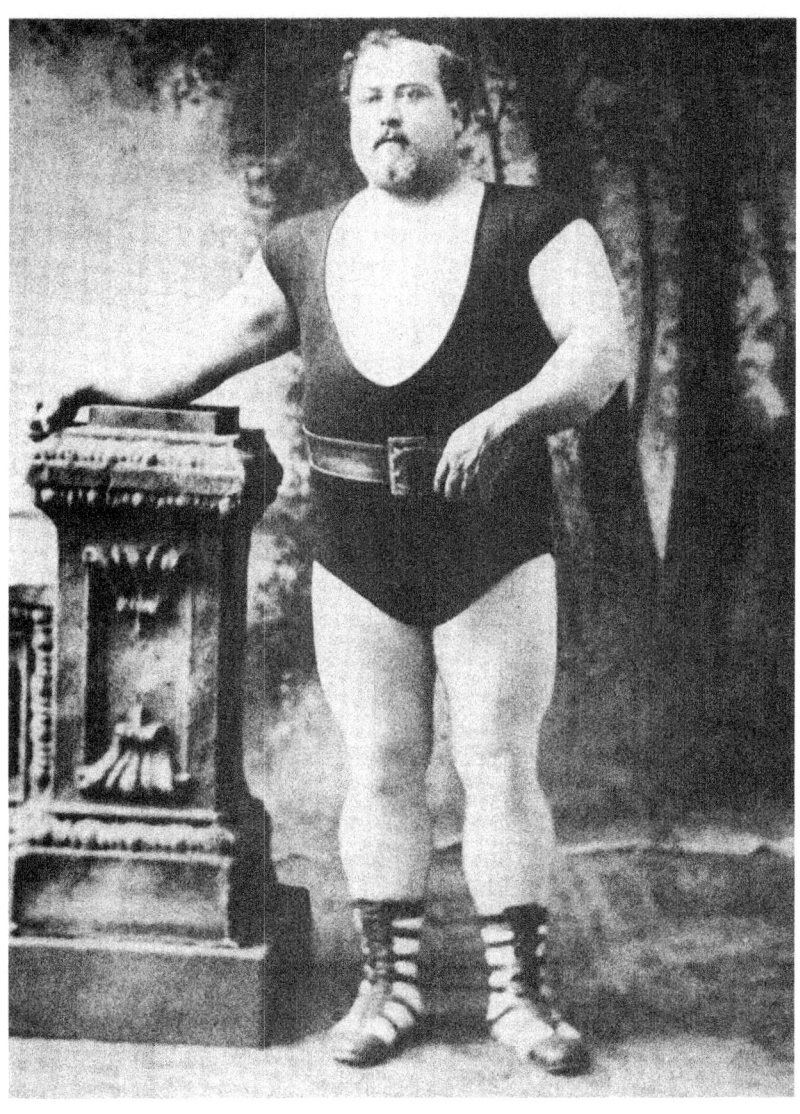

Figure 13.5 The great Louis Cyr.

For many, this way of thinking will require a change of attitude. It will make it necessary to embrace one's body type and natural inclination, and to develop a sense of confidence in it, or, rather, in the *abilities* of one's body as opposed to its *visual appearance*. It will make it necessary to acknowledge that oldtime strongmen came in various appearances and body types, and that anyone can fall in the category of "oldtime strong-man" if he is able to *do* with his body the things oldtime strongman did.

For example, if you are of the *brawny* type but have a little belly, as opposed to visually separated abdominal muscles, and in theory have the ability to get rid of this belly with dieting and lots of cardiovascular exercise, but accompanied by a considerable decrease in your maximum strength, you might want to determine that this *you* with visible abdominal muscles is simply *not* you. Thus, adopt a positive way of thinking in the sense of focusing on what you *are* instead of what you *are not*. Your defining assets are that you are a *big, massive, broad-shouldered,* and *strong* fellow. It is a waste of time and energy to focus on the fact that you *are not* ripped, just as you *are not* blond or red-haired, for example.

The opposite is true if you are of the *wiry* body type, but crave a higher body weight, greater muscle mass, and thicker arms and legs. If you force yourself to eat at least six high-caloric meals per day, consuming part of these meals in liquid form, and consciously restrict your weekly hours of exercise, you might be able to gain some weight and muscle mass. However, as a side effect you will also gain some body fat, and lose your asset of being a wiry fellow with visibly cut muscles. You might end up with mediocre muscle mass and mediocre muscle definition, as your natural inclination does not favour the above-average muscle mass you crave. Here, one might ask whether it were not wiser to proudly embrace the fact that you are wiry and cut. You could take advantage of this through the element of surprise – doing feats that much bigger fellows can not – or focusing on feats like the one-arm pull-up, for example, which you could never do with a higher body weight.

While I firmly believe that an attitude like the above will greatly benefit both your strength aims and peace of mind, I need to mention two aspects that relativize this to a certain degree:

Aspect 1): It is more easily possible to change your body type considerably by the use of performance-enhancing drugs. However, I believe this is the exception that proves my rule best, because, as commonly known, the use of performance-enhancing drugs bears great risks to your overall health, and thus takes its toll in a different area – not even taking into account for now that oldtime strongman training and performance-enhancing drugs do generally not go together very well.

Aspect 2): If you are either of the *wiry* or *overweight* body type, not because of a natural inclination, but because of unhealthy living conditions and nutrition habits, you might want to consider a change to your lifestyle and diet after all – not primarily to improve your looks, but to increase your overall health. If, for example, you are of the *overweight* type because you lead a sedentary lifestyle, and your nutrition regularly consists of the disgusting processed foods that are advertised by some of the common and famous brand names, you might want to consider switching to a proper diet (ideally a "Görner Diet", as I will explain below in the corresponding chapter), and taking up the habit of regular long forest walks in the fresh air. By these comparatively small efforts you will perhaps automatically discover that your natural inclination is in fact the *brawny* type.

The same is true if you believe that you belong to the *wiry* type, which you deduce must be equivalent to the *"pale* and *sickly"* type. Incidentally, you lead a purely indoor and solitary lifestyle, shun sunlight for fear of sunburn, and contact with other living beings for fear of bacteria. You follow a diet that consists first and foremost of sugared and caffeinated liquids, because you are – by natural inclination, it seems – not blessed with an appetite for solid foods. Instead, you are blessed with the properties of a so-called night owl, who stays up late, and solves computational riddles all night long. If this is the case, you might want to question whether this condition, your modest physical substance, light skin, and lack of appetite, might not be connected to your lifestyle as well. Who knows whether you would not fare better if you began spending some hours of the day outdoors, began building a properly operating immune system by getting into contact with nature and other human beings, began getting an adequate amount of quality sleep, and began eating some real and tasty foods, like farm-fresh sauerkraut, wholemeal *Pumpernickel* bread, or free-range eggs from chicken who have seen the sunlight.

If one or more of these aspects apply to you, you should utilize the power of *habit*. Force yourself to make these changes, until they become habits and no longer require a conscious effort – just like your unhealthy lifestyle was a habit until now, albeit a *bad* habit.

Having mentioned these important aspects, I nevertheless want to give some input to those who will not discard the idea that they have to change their body type, not for health reasons, but to accommodate a certain *idea* of how they believe they are *supposed* to look if they want to call themselves oldtime strongmen.

Although I said above that there is no such thing as *the* look of the oldtime strongman, there are some particularities that differentiated these men visually from most modern-day trainees, strength athletes, or bodybuilders. As I already mentioned earlier, two weightlifting exercises that are rather common today, were virtually unknown in the golden age of the strongman, *viz.* the back squat and the bench press. Therefore, one should believe that these men tended to have narrower thighs and smaller chests than the average (serious) modern-day trainee. However, some of the oldtime strongmen nevertheless managed to build huge thighs. They did so, either through all their cleans, overhead-, back-, and harness lifting, or because they were generally versatile athletes who were sprinters, jumpers, or wrestlers at the same time as they were weightlifters.

Talking about wrestling: in my opinion, the famous wrestler George Hackenschmidt had the best-developed physique of the golden age and was the one oldtime strongman who came closest to the look of a modern-day bodybuilder, including his leg development. At least I have never seen a photograph of anyone from the golden age with a better physical development. Mind you that the invention of the "Hackenschmidt squat" is attributed to George Hackenschmidt. This was originally a barbell exercise very different to the modern Hackenschmidt *machines*. It resembled a deadlift with the barbell behind one's feet and legs.

With regard to chest development, I should say that yes, on average, the oldtime strongmen had smaller chests. But in my opinion, this was not necessarily a bad thing, as most will agree that the over-developed chests of some modern-day trainees are often on the brink of grotesqueness and out of proportion with the rest of their bodies.

Furthermore, the oldtime strongmen, although being able and strong overhead lifters, lacked the kind of shoulder and trapezius muscle development that even amateur bodybuilders boast today. The reason for this is that they did not use any of the performance-enhancing drugs that are so popular in our modern times, like artificial testosterone hormones. Such substances have the effect of causing a disproportionate growth of the neck and shoulder muscles, which does not necessarily need to be connected to an intense training of these.

As a side note, it is a commonly known fact that the *natural* testosterone in all men of our so-called Western civilization is gradually decreasing since several generations, for reasons still not entirely clear. Therefore, the oldtime strongmen on average must surely have had more *natural* testosterone on average than modern men. However, I suspect that this difference is still comparatively small, as it does not seem to have caused the kind of well-rounded and protruding shoulder and trapezius muscles as in the substance-using athletes of our modern days.

Last but not least, because of the feats oldtime strongmen trained for, they typically had strong tendons and ligaments. These favour a look of thick joints and forearms. A large amount of grip and wrist training, e.g. with steel bending training, and/or physical work, develops thick forearms in some athletes (although one can have a very strong grip without necessarily having thick forearms – it is a common misconception that there exists a direct relation between the two). The best example is probably the Canadian oldtime strongman Arthur Dandurand, whose disproportionally thick right forearm leaves any modern beholder of his photographs awestruck.

In conclusion, if one wanted to acquire a typical oldtime strongman look, he should first of all embrace his body type, and not try to change it. Within these boundaries, he should lift lots of heavy weights, refrain from too much bench pressing, and perform lots of exercises that stress tendons and ligaments, like heavy grip, wrist, and forearm training. In essence, one should perform an oldtime strongman *training routine* to acquire the oldtime strongman *look*. With this insight I have come full circle to demonstrate the absurdity of training *for* an oldtime strongman look. For some of the strongest oldtime strongmen, *looks* were the result of their *training*, rather than their *training* a result of their *desired looks*. There are exceptions to this rule, of course, like the German oldtime strongmen and bodybuilders Eugene Sandow and Lionel Strongfort, who took great pride in their visual muscular development.

All of this being said, there are two basic ways in which you can change your physical appearance: either by gaining muscle mass or by losing body-fat. With the right information and a certain amount of discipline, both are actually not that difficult to achieve. What is difficult, however, is to do both at the same time. In particular, it is difficult to make great progress in both within a *short period of time*. It also requires a great effort to *maintain* both great muscle mass and a low body-fat percentage at the same time. Therefore, to make your life easier and leave enough room for you to keep focused on your strength goals, I strongly suggest you try to do one thing at a time: Either try to build muscle mass or try to lose body-fat.

In addition to this, you always have a third option: to not worry about looks at all, but focus on your strength goals only. In sum, you have three different goals that you can focus on temporarily (but not simultaneously):

1. Build muscle mass
2. Gain strength
3. Reduce body-fat

If you do care about looks *and* strength, I suggest you design your nutrition and training according to a cycle that takes these three goals into consideration one after the other. For instance, you can have a yearly cycle that focuses on one of these goals during a predetermined number of months.

Here is an example:

- ◆ January: gain strength
- ◆ February: gain strength
- ◆ March: reduce body-fat
- ◆ April: reduce body-fat
- ◆ May: reduce body-fat
- ◆ June: reduce body-fat
- ◆ July: build muscle mass
- ◆ August: build muscle mass
- ◆ September: build muscle mass
- ◆ October: build muscle mass
- ◆ November: gain strength
- ◆ December: gain strength

In the example above, you dedicate four months per year to one of the three goals. You start dieting roughly when the Christian Lent starts, to make sure you look good when summer comes. In the middle of summer, when you start feeling skinny, you switch to a muscle-mass building plan. In the cold and dark winter months, when you have built some substance, you care about nothing but strength any more.

I have made good experiences with such a cycle, especially because it reduces boredom, and also because I believe it is quite natural and healthy for the human body to go from periods of plenty to periods of fasting, cyclically and according to the seasons (although traditionally, the winter months were probably the "dieting" months). Four months per goal is also an ample period of time to make good progress.

But however you decide to arrange your yearly cycle is up to you. You can reduce or increase the number of months you dedicate to one goal – for example, diet for only two months per year – or adapt your yearly cycle to the specific date of an upcoming competition. Incidentally, as you might know, most professional bodybuilders also work with such cycles and periods of dieting before an important competition.

Most of this book is already dedicated to the question of how you should train (and eat) to gain strength. So let me now talk shortly about how you should adapt both training and nutrition for the other two goals: building muscle mass and losing body-fat. In general, the rules and principles I establish in this book, should be equally applied to the periods dedicated to these latter two goals. It would not be a good idea to completely change your workout plan during your mass building and dieting seasons, or leave out all your specialized strength-building exercises completely.

This would make it much harder for you to get back on track in your strength season. Keep in mind, however, that minor strength losses are inevitable and quite normal during a dieting season, and can usually be compensated for in your strength season. Ideally, you take one step back and two steps forward, so to say.

Also, you can apply the principle of variation in accordance with your cycle, and try different exercises, or leave others out temporarily. But keep your ultimate strength goals in mind. Likewise, a proper "Görner Diet" (see below), with some adaptations that I will explain in the following, is best for all three seasons and necessary to ensure you get all the essential nutrients.

Here are some suggestions for your *muscle-building* season, which, if obeyed, will increase your muscle mass effectively. All of them are meant as *changes* to your *standard situation* or *condition*, where you neither gain nor lose weight:

1. Reduce your general *physical activity*. Walk when you would run, stand when you would walk, sit when you would stand, and lie when you would sit.
2. Reduce the *number* of workouts per week (the absolute minimum is two) and reduce the *duration* of your workouts (the absolute minimum is 45 minutes).
3. (And thus increase the *periods of rest* between workouts.)
4. But: increase the *intensity* of your workouts. Go (close to) to your limit in every working set.
5. Perform *heavy, compound exercises*, like squats, shoulder press, bench press, barbell rows, deadlifts, pull-ups, etc.
6. Perform your working sets with about *eight to ten* repetitions per set.
7. Increase the *number* of meals per day, or add snacks in between your meals.
8. Increase the *amount* of food you eat per meal.
9. Especially increase the *amount of protein* you eat.
10. Increase the amount of *caloric-dense* foods, like nuts, legumes, healthy fats, etc.

These ten simple measures will have the logical consequence that your muscle mass will increase (given a certain number of general prerequisites, like an adequate amount of sleep, proper execution of the weightlifting exercises, overall health, intake of all essential nutrients, and so on).

And here are some rules to follow if you want to *reduce your body-fat* effectively:

1. Increase your general *physical activity*. Run when you would walk, walk when you would stand, stand when you would sit, sit when you would lie (except in bed during the nights).
2. Increase the *number* of workouts per week (the absolute maximum is six) and increase the *duration* of your workouts (the absolute maximum is two hours).
3. Add some *cardiovascular training* to your weightlifting training, like swimming, running, hiking, or cycling.
4. Maintain a *mediocre intensity* of your weightlifting workouts.
5. But: *increase* the number of exercises you perform per workout, *increase* the number of sets you perform per exercise, and *reduce* the pauses between the sets.
6. Perform your working sets with about *ten to fifteen* repetitions per set.
7. Keep your *number* of meals per day high.
8. But: Reduce the *amount* of food you eat per meal.
9. Keep the *amount of protein* you eat high.
10. Increase the amount of *low-caloric* foods you eat, and there is only one type of true low-caloric foods: vegetables.
11. But: reduce either your *fat intake* of your *carbohydrate intake* drastically. Both methods have been proven to work (I prefer to reduce my carbohydrate intake).

It is really as simple as that, but it is important not to be in a hurry with either goal. If you track your progress too impatiently, this will inevitably lead to frustration and ill-considered action, like giving up your plan altogether or falling prey to the empty promises and proclaimed rocket science of the countless diet gurus out there. Especially when you start a diet, it can take some time for your body to adapt to your new "lifestyle". I would say after about two weeks you will be adequately used to it. You might also want to make this transition step by step and smoothly, e.g. by cutting your carbohydrate intake in the first week, taking up cardiovascular activity in the second week, etc. In this way it will not be such a shock for your body and psyche, and easier to pull through.

Although I believe that a healthy body should have an adequate amount of muscle tissue and a low to moderate body-fat percentage, there is a certain paradox in *acquiring* both. It is neither healthy to radically increase your muscle mass, nor to diet. For these reasons, you will probably not *feel best* during either of these phases, which is quite logic if you look at it from the following perspective: The force-feeding and the lazy lifestyle of your muscle-building phase are quite obviously not healthy. But dieting puts the body in a state of want. If you effectively lose body-fat and thus body weight, your body obviously burns more of its substance than it gets back through nutrition, which is a condition of depletion. If continued endlessly, it would eventually lead to starvation, which is not considered healthy either (although some people argue that fasting, for example, is quite natural and even healthy for the body – but only over limited periods of time).

You will probably feel best when your strength season comes, when you simply get involved in the type and amount of activity you enjoy, and eat the amounts of food your body dictates (remember that your body usually takes what it needs automatically). Keep this in mind during your muscle-building and dieting phases and do not overdo it.

14. Putting it all together: Designing your workouts and devising a plan

I have now introduced you to a lot of different principles, concepts, and techniques to build oldtime strength. Which of these you implement in your training, and how, depends on a lot of different factors, including your immediate and long-term goals, prior experience, priorities, preferences, and personality. You might either want to train for one or two specific feats of strength I have introduced, you might want to perform oldtime strongman training simply for fitness purposes or for a different sport you play, you might want to live a complete oldtime strongman lifestyle, or you might be thinking about stepping on a stage to do an oldtime strongman performance. You might have zero experience with strength training whatsoever, you might be an avid weightlifter, bodybuilder, or powerlifter who wants to specialize, or you might be a professional athlete in a different kind of sport. You might be young, independent and flexible, or you might be married with children and working 60 hours per week in a strenuous job.

Depending on your individual situation, you will hopefully pick out the information from this book that suits you best, and design your workouts accordingly. Nevertheless, I want to give you a short summary of the most important concepts I introduced, and some general ideas of how they can be combined and implemented into an efficient workout plan.

The concepts that I have introduced so far, and that you might want to consider, include:

1. The human movement patterns
2. Training for overall body strength
3. How to decide which strongman feats suit you
4. The general principles of training for oldtime strongman feats
5. Categorization of specific strongman feats and specialized training for such
6. The concept of specialization or setting priorities in training
7. The concept of changing one's focus over longer periods of time

To recapitulate and put this in a simple form, when you devise your oldtime strongman training plan, I recommend that you, in your training:

1. Cover all of the basic human movement patterns in one way or another
2. Make sure that you train for an adequate amount of overall body strength (according to the movement patterns)

3. Make a (first) decision of which (category/ies of) strongman feats you want to train for
4. Heed the general principles of *progression, continuity, variation,* and *partialisation*
5. Devise a specialized training regimen for the (category/ies of) feat(s) of strength of your choice
6. Stick to this specialized training regimen for this/these (category/ies of) feat(s) for an adequate amount of time
7. Adapt your focus according to age

To avoid that you do not see the wood for the trees, I think two examples will illustrate best what I mean. Let us assume there is an aspiring oldtime strongman with the following profile:

♦ Age: 20 years old
♦ Size: 90kg (199lbs) bodyweight, 185cm (6ft) height
♦ Family status: bachelor
♦ Job: carpenter
♦ Experience: former wrestler
♦ Interest: a broad and varied oldtime strongman training routine
♦ Goal: overall oldtime strength, only for private purposes and fun

This young man has lots of possibilities and great prerequisites for building oldtime strength. At 20 years of age, he is still in his prime and can tackle a high work load in his training, as well as complex, taxing exercises – even such that require explosive strength. His bodyweight in relation to his height demonstrates that he is neither the wiry nor the overweight type, but still has some potential to gain muscle and become a strongman of the brawny type. Some more substance could help him with heavy natural stone lifting, for example. On the positive side, his job and prior experience as a wrestler will have conditioned his muscles, bones, and ligaments to a large degree, and thus created ideal prerequisites to becoming a strongman. On the negative side, his body will already have experienced some trauma and tear and wear, and his strenuous job will claim some of his energy every day.

Let us look at his interests and goals: The athlete is open to general oldtime strongman training, rather than only one particular feat. Combining this fact with his age and body type, he certainly has the potential to approach feats like overhead strength and stone lifting, so I would put an initial focus on these, with lots of deadlifts and shoulder presses. I would also put a secondary focus on grip strength and wrist strength, as these are of utmost importance in oldtime strongman training. He is not interested in performances, so there is no need to train for feats that are mostly designed for show purposes, like teeth strength feats.

Before I suggest an individual workout plan for this imaginary person, let me cover a few basic aspects that apply to any type of strength training (to many of my readers this will already be common knowledge and they can skip the following section). Some of these I have already mentioned:

♦ A good number of workouts per week is three to five
♦ Any workout should be preceded by a general and specific warm-up
♦ A good duration of a day's workout (including warm-up) is between one and two hours
♦ A day's workout consists of several exercises, which are typically performed several times with breaks in between. One of these is called a set and typically consists of several repetitions (sometimes this is just one repetition)
♦ A good rule of thumb for strength training is to perform between three to five sets per exercise and between two to six repetitions per set
♦ The break between two sets, whether of the same or different exercises, should be between one and five minutes, i.e. not too long and not too short

Based on this, here is a suggestion for a workout plan for the athlete introduced above:

Monday: "Lifting and carrying" and "dexterity I"/Stone lifting training
♦ Thick bar deadlifts for grip strength and to warm-up for:
♦ Heavy deadlifts (replace every few weeks by trying to lift and carry *challenge stone*)
♦ Heavy barbell rows
♦ Lifting *training stone* for repetitions
♦ Carrying *training stone* for distance

Tuesday: "Throwing"/Overhead training
♦ Heavy military shoulder press
♦ Heavy barbell push press
♦ Heavy dumbbell push press
♦ Dumbbell flies on bench
♦ Kettlebell juggling

167

Wednesday: Rest day

Thursday: "Climbing" and "dexterity II"
- Pull-ups on fingertips
- Heavy barbell curls
- Wrist curls
- Reverse wrist curls
- Sledgehammer levering

Friday: "Walking, running, and jumping", "hitting" and "biting"
- Squats
- Front squats
- Stiff-legged deadlifts
- Various abdominal exercises
- Wrestler's bridges

Saturday & Sunday: Rest day

This is a tough workout plan that trains the whole body and includes lots of heavy compound exercises. It will be very strenuous, but doable for a natural 20-year-old athlete, considering that there are three rest days per week. It puts a great focus on the movement patterns and muscle groups required for heavy natural stone lifting: back, biceps, grip, wrists, and so on. For the throwing movement pattern, it puts more emphasis on shoulder exercises than chest exercises, to be in accordance with the oldtime spirit, but also because the athlete might also want to lift the one or the other stone overhead. Nevertheless, it contains a dedicated chest exercise, dumbbell flies, which build some of the strength for the "hugging" of heavy stones. The regimen contains a leg day, which is also designed to help with the stone lifting, as it contains front squats and stiff-legged deadlifts. The amount of grip- and wrist strength training is limited, but complete. It will prepare the athlete in case he wants to change his focus to steel bending and specialized grip strength feats later in his life. As he has no ambitions to train for teeth strength, he does some wrestler's bridges, which he is already familiar with from his earlier wrestling training.

Let us analyse this regimen by asking some questions:

1. Does the workout plan cover all of the basic human movement patterns in one way or another? Yes, it does. There is "walking, running, and jumping", "throwing", "climbing", "lifting and carrying", "hitting", "biting", and "dexterity".

2. Does it make sure he trains for an adequate amount of overall body strength (according to the movement patterns)? Yes, it does, as it contains lots of basic compound exercises like deadlifts, overhead presses, squats, and pull-ups, although the athlete already has an amount of overall body strength from his wrestling training and work on construction sites.

3. Has the athlete made a (first) decision of which (category/ies of) strongman feats he wants to train for? Yes, he has: stone lifting and overhead lifting.

4. Does he heed the general principles of *progression, continuity, variation*, and *partialisation*? Cannot tell from looking at the workout plan, but hopefully, yes. He should regularly try to increase the weight and/or repetitions in each exercise, try to lift his training stone for more repetitions, and try to carry it further. He should vary his grip position from time to time when he does pull-ups on his finger tips, and he should experiment with his technique when lifting/carrying his stones. Yes, he applies the principle of partialisation, as he performs exercises that will assist him in the various phases of lifting natural stones (deadlifts, barbell rows, front squats, dumbbell flies, wrist curls...).

5. Has he devised a specialized training regimen for the (category/ies of) feat(s) of strength of his choice? Yes, he has. Everything in his workout plan fits well together to cover all movement patterns, yet almost every workout day feeds into his ambitions with natural stone lifting. He performs heavy barbell exercises that build the muscles required for stone lifting *and* trains with actual stones.

6. Does he stick to this specialized training regimen for this/these (category/ies of) feat(s) for an adequate amount of time? Cannot tell from looking at the regimen, but he should definitely stick to this plan for at least a year to make reasonable progress.

7. Does he adapt his focus according to age? Yes, as a rather young athlete he has made his choice to train for two more difficult and compound categories of oldtime strongman feats, which are stone lifting and overhead lifting. Yet, he paves his way to taking up grip strength and bending feats later on, as he already includes exercises to condition his muscles and ligaments for such.

I hope you understand what I mean and how my principles can be applied when devising a workout plan.

Let me now give you another example, an imaginary workout plan for the following athlete:

- ◆ Age: 35 years old
- ◆ Size: 78kg (172lbs) bodyweight, 182cm (5ft 11in) height
- ◆ Family status: married, two children
- ◆ Job: accountant
- ◆ Experience: some track and field training in his youth; lifelong interest in endurance sports, regularly runs half-marathons; general training with weights since ten years, has attended some power-lifting meets for fun. Best raw lifts: 160kg (353lbs) squat, 110kg (243lbs) bench press, 200kg (442lbs) deadlift.
- ◆ Interest: grip and steel bending
- ◆ Goal: attend grip strength contests, bend the Ironmind Red Nail

This gentleman is considerably older than the first, but still at an age where he can make great progress in terms of strength, and even, with some effort, "oldtime strength". Luckily, he has lots of experience in different sports, and thus a good all-round foundation, although he does not truly excel at any specific discipline. His powerlifting performance is not out of the ordinary so far, but sufficient to build on, and greater lifting ability is not necessary to capitalize on grip and bending strength.

Judging from his height and weight, and his ability to run half-marathons at a regular rate, combined with his nevertheless considerable overall strength, he appears to me as a typical representative of the wiry type: good muscular development, low body fat, and relatively small frame. If I were him, I would not force myself into trying to become a different body type, for example by trying to gain a large amount of muscle mass. This is not necessary for grip and steel bending strength. As an accountant, he is lucky that he can channel all his physical energy into his workouts, but since he also has a family and full-time job, his time and mental energy are limited. He has no interest in performing feats of strength in front of an audience, but he wants to attend grip strength contests and wants to certify for a recognized feat of strength.

Here is my suggestion for a workout plan:

Monday: "Running, and jumping", "dexterity 1", and "hitting"
- Squat
- Sledgehammer levering
- Wrist curls
- Reverse wrist curls
- Sledgehammer swings

Tuesday: Rest day

Wednesday: "Throwing"
- Bench Press
- Steel bending training
- Narrow-grip bench press

Thursday: Rest day

Friday: "Lifting and carrying", "dexterity 2", and "climbing"
- Deadlifts
- Hand gripper training
- Thick bar lifts
- Pinch grip exercises
- Pull-ups (optional: on fingertips, with thick bar, or on slings of rope with limited number of fingers, etc.)

Saturday & Sunday: "Walking"
- Endurance sports like running, hiking, cycling...

To start with, I have reduced the workload of this athlete to three days per week, as he is very busy in his job and needs to spend time with his family. Also, at 35, he needs more recovery time than a 20-year-old. Three days of training per week make it possible for him to have at least one day of recovery before each day of training. As he is already used to a powerlifting routine, I would let him retain this and start each of his three trainings with one of the powerlifting moves (no assistance exercises, though), to maintain, or build, overall body strength. Thus, he can get these moves "over with" early in his trainings and his body his well warmed-up when he approaches his specialized grip and bending training. Each day contains an aspect of this:

On Mondays, he does his squats, and trains his wrists in all directions – starting with sledgehammer levering for nail bending in particular. The workout closes with sledgehammer swings for the abdominal muscles, because he already has the hammer at hand, and because this is also a great conditioning exercise for the hands.

Wednesdays begin with the bench press, which strengthens the chest, and is therefore beneficial for his steel bending training. Next comes one of the climaxes of his training week: his actual steel bending training with nails, horseshoes, steel bars, or whatever. To wrap this training up, he does some narrow-grip bench presses to strengthen his triceps, as triceps strength helps in many steel bending feats.

Fridays begin with regular deadlifts, perhaps not too heavy (to conserve enough energy for the specialized grip strength training) but heavy enough to be well warmed-up. He should not spend too much time on his deadlift training, to have enough time left for the second climax of his training week: his specialized grip strength training with hand gripper training, thick bar lifts, and pinch grip exercises. With these he can go wild, experiment, and play around with variations of the many different grip strength exercises that exist. I have placed hand gripper training first, as I assume this is his priority, but if a thick bar or pinch grip feat is his priority at the moment, he should perform these exercises first. The training closes with pull-ups, to maintain general strength in the back and biceps muscles, and to stretch his spine after the deadlifts and thick bar lifts. On this day, he also has the option to focus even more by turning the deadlifts and/or pull-ups into grip strength exercises, and doing only specialized grip strength exercises for the feat he is focusing on at the moment. For example, if he is currently training for a pinch grip feat, he could do his deadlifts with a limited number of fingers, like two fingers or one finger per hand, do his pull-ups on a (revolving) thick bar, and do only pinch grip exercises in his specialized training (and have no dynamic grip strength exercises, like hand gripper training, for the moment).

Let us now analyse this workout schedule with the seven questions from above:

1. Does the workout plan cover all of the basic human movement patterns in one way or another? Yes, it does. There is "walking" at the weekend, in the form of endurance sports, there is "running and jumping", "throwing", "climbing", "lifting and carrying", "hitting", and "dexterity". There is no "biting" training, as he has no ambition to perform or train teeth strength feats.

However, his nutrition regularly includes raw vegetables and is generally rich in fibre.

2. Does it make sure he trains for an adequate amount of overall body strength (according to the movement patterns)? Yes, it does, as it contains the three powerlifting moves, pull-ups, and sledgehammer swings, which cover the most important basic movement patterns in addition to his specialized training.

3. Has he made a (first) decision of which (category/ies of) strongman feats he wants to train for? Yes, he has: nail bending and grip strength. These combine well as they benefit from each other.

4. Does he heed the general principles of *progression, continuity, variation*, and *partialisation*? Cannot tell from looking at the workout plan, but hopefully, yes. He should regularly try to increase the weight and/or repetitions in each grip strength and wrist strength exercise, and try to progress to tougher nails, or the same nails reduced in length. Likewise, he should try to close his challenge hand gripper with the handle farther and farther apart. He should vary his grip exercises to prepare for a diversified grip strength contest and he should experiment with his technique when nail bending. Yes, he applies the principle of partialisation, as he performs exercises that will assist him in the various phases of steel bending (wrist strength, chest strength, triceps strength...).

5. Has he devised a specialized training regimen for the (category/ies of) feat(s) of strength of his choice? Yes, he has. On each of his three training days, specialized wrist or grip training is the main focus, while training for overall body strength is reduced to a minimum.

6. Does he stick to this specialized training regimen for this/these (category/ies of) feat(s) for an adequate amount of time? Cannot tell from looking at the regimen, but he should definitely stick to this plan for at least a year to make reasonable progress.

7. Does he adapt his focus according to age? Yes, as a middle-aged athlete he has chosen a focus where he can still make great progress.

15. Your body is part of the equation as well

I have already touched upon the issue of health and I have also hinted at the fact that your body is not indestructible. Without wanting to leave my readers overly pessimistic, I believe one should not ignore these facts of life. One cannot talk about heavy oldtime strongman training and all those fantastic strength gains, without mentioning that *your body is part of the equation as well*. What I mean is, you should take good care of your body and health, to make strength gains and to be able to keep up an intense oldtime strongman training routine.

If you have a good and expensive pair of leather shoes that you want to keep for a long time, I suppose you brush it when it is dirty, you shine it regularly, you stuff it out with newspaper when it gets wet, and you give it to your trusted shoemaker to replace the sole when it is broken. Just as you take care of such a good pair of shoes you want to keep for a long time, you should take good care of your body if you want it to perform well for a long time. Even more so since your body cannot be replaced like a pair of shoes, and since it is much more difficult to change parts of it that are broken (although this is possible to a certain degree with modern medicine).

Thus, just as you clean, shine, and care for your shoes, you should take care of your hygiene, nutrition, and general health. Your body is your most important tool, and in case you make money with strongman performances, it is nothing less but your *capital*. You should therefore be aware of how you treat your body, what you feed it, and the signals it gives you.

What is good (and bad) for the body? Although you will hear lots of different answers to this question, depending on whom you ask, I know the true answer, as it is actually quite simple. In fact, we all know what is good for our body, but most of us lack the discipline to do these things. As for myself, ever since I earn money with oldtime strongman performances, it has helped me tremendously to perceive my body as my capital. I thus have a *duty* to always do what is best for my body, because otherwise I would increase the risk of losing part of my income (a risk that is high enough already), which I need to feed my family. With this kind of attitude I always have a good excuse to *restrain* from things that are bad for my health and body, and to *do* the things that are good. These things I will illustrate in the following.

Things that are bad for health and body:

♦ Psychological stress
♦ Alcohol
♦ Smoking
♦ Unhealthy food
♦ A sedentary lifestyle
♦ Overweight
♦ Injuries
♦ Toxic substances

Things that are good for health and body:

♦ A healthy nutrition
♦ Long nights of good sleep
♦ Great amounts of light, natural movement across all joints of the body
♦ Periods of rest and reflection
♦ Peace of mind
♦ Meaningful relationships and social interaction
♦ Proper hygiene
♦ Clean and fresh air
♦ A certain amount of sunlight

Below, I have included a separate chapter on nutrition, in which I will talk in detail about food. As to the other aspects listed above, I will give you a few general pieces of advice here. Most of these should already be common knowledge, but lots of people still disregard them, in the belief that they are unable to change anything about their lives – either because they do not feel self-determined, or because they do not believe they have the power and discipline to alter their own habits. I believe in many cases, it is simply choices one has to make, as I will explain below.

I think *psychological stress* is one of the biggest factors that can inhibit your training success. Fear of job loss, time management problems, relationship problems, an overload of work... All of these things cost a lot of energy – energy that could be mobilized in your training instead. Lots of people in our time have to deal with such problems, and this would not be the case if there were an easy solution to this. Thus, I will not pretend that I have one.

However, I believe one thing that could help, would be to structure, minimize, and clear up your life – to remove as much "clutter" as you can. If your room or house is a mess – clean it up. If you find little time for the pleasant things in life – structure your day and stick to it. Make a place for time with your spouse, with your children, for housework, to relax, to let your mind wander, etc. Review your to-do-list and delete unnecessary items. Do the same with your material belongings and relationships. And, of course, make a place for training time. When this time comes, train free from guilt. It is all a matter of choice. Do you choose to set so many goals that you feel overwhelmed all the time and that your to-do-list is constantly full? Do you choose to purchase an item you do not really need, which will clutter your home and cost you money you have spent so much time on to earn? And so on.

Alcohol and *smoking* are two big health risks that everyone is aware of, but those who regularly indulge in them cannot seem to give them up. Even if you do not indulge in drinks and cigarettes to a high degree, remember that you always have the option of limiting your intake even more. Refraining from smoking and drinking can reduce the vast majority of relevant health risks in our society. And it is very easy to say no when you are aware that it does nothing good to your body. This is a question of inner conviction. Then, it is just a choice you have to make, either one big choice, like saying, "I am a non-smoker," or lots of little choices, like, "Today, I will have a non-alcoholic drink."

The same is true of a *sedentary lifestyle*: The habit of sitting too many hours per day is one of the big factors that cause all sorts of health issues in our society. Everybody knows, but everybody has a hard time trying to do something against it. Sitting is just so comfortable. Try to turn this around and develop an attitude that *walking* is good for your body. Do not be annoyed by the fact that you have to get up from your seat ever so often, but embrace the fact! Spring to your feet gladly and full of energy, to get a cup of coffee, to talk to a colleague, or to fetch your mail. Rush up the stairs energetically, take two or three steps at a time, and rejoice in the fact that you can. All of these little steps (in a literal sense) add up throughout the day.

Overweight as a health risk is equally well known, and this can be an issue to aspiring strongmen who aim to build a large amount of muscle mass. Of course, muscle is better than body fat, but being heavy either way contains all sorts of issues – independent of the distribution of this weight: Greater body mass causes greater stress on your joints, digestion problems, circulatory problems, and so on. I believe that much of your body composition is dictated by your natural constitution. But even so, mind you that some oldtime strongmen have actually been rather small and wiry fellows, with incredible strength nevertheless. You do not have to be a second Emil Naucke.

You must have wondered why I list such an obvious fact as *injuries* as something that is bad for your body. One would think everybody tries to avoid injuries naturally, but this is not the case. You can reduce the risk of

177

injuries in many different ways, and again I will leave it up to you to make the choice or not. For example, you can reduce the risk of injury by refraining from activities that are fast or high – car racing, motorcycling, skiing, climbing, parachuting, etc. Refraining from the intake of performance-enhancing drugs reduces the risk of lifting heavy weights your muscles can move, but your tendons and ligaments are not ready for yet (remember that these take much more time to grow and adapt). Being impatient and reckless can also lead to injuries, and it is your choice to behave in such a way, or be wise and considerate.

One aspect I believe many strength enthusiasts disregard in our times, although it gets more and more attention in the media, is the amount of *toxic substances* we feed into our body, directly and indirectly, throughout the day. People become increasingly aware that all sorts of substances in foods, grooming products, healthcare products, clothes, and products of everyday use, can potentially harm the human body. The amount of products contaminated in this way appears to be so high that it seems impossible to avoid the direct and indirect consumption of such. However, one can at least make an effort to avoid such toxins wherever possible. A simple way to do so is a sort of traditionalism combined with minimalism. It helps to imagine the world as it was 150 years ago, and perceive some aspects of life as if we were still living in these times, as I will explain in the following. I am not saying that the world has not changed for the better since then, and some of the modern innovations should be embraced for their potential to alleviate suffering and trouble in the world. But in many other areas of daily life we would do ourselves something good if we lived our everyday lives as we did a long time ago.

One example is *food*. Although I will talk more about food later, I should mention here that if you have the possibility, you should source your food locally and according to the seasons, eating those vegetables and fruit that are harvested at a particular time of the year. But let us not anticipate too much with regard to food yet.

In terms of *grooming products*, a simpler, naturally produced, and traditionally crafted source is often the better choice than some of the modern products. The latter often contain large amounts of chemicals and substances whose true impact on the body is not sufficiently known. Such modern products might "do their job" exceptionally well, for example to achieve a certain cosmetic result, but what is the point if they harm your body at the same time? In most cases, simple, natural, traditional, and locally sourced products are sufficient.

I do by no means want to talk you out of using modern *healthcare products* if you have a medical condition. I believe we should be grateful for the advancements in modern medicine. However, as some of these products also contain large amounts of toxic substances, I personally try to use them only when really necessary. Once a certain illness is cured, I try to analyse what caused the illness in the first place, how it could have been avoided, and how I can avoid it in the future. But I will talk more about healthcare below.

With regard to *clothes*, I try to wear items of natural textiles and avoid those consisting of the modern, artificial materials. But even textiles of a natural origin, like cotton, contain lots of toxic substances these days, including herbicides, pesticides, and in particular dyes. In addition to this, it is almost impossible to efficiently trace the source of the material you are wearing. Especially new products seem to contain large amounts of harmful substances, which are washed out only gradually over time. It therefore seems to be a good idea to keep and use your clothes for as long as possible – assuming that your older clothes contain less chemicals. Maintain, repair, and wear your clothes for as long as you can. This will save you money, and there is nothing shabby about it, because you owe it to the environment and the people who produced your clothes to value them.

For the same reasons, I try to avoid clothing that corresponds to a current, fast-lived fashion. Such pieces will be out of fashion just as fast, forcing you to buy new items over and over again. Instead of this foolish procedure, I would suggest going for a classic, timeless style. In particular if you are a gentleman, this is an easy thing to do. Classic men's fashion changes only very slowly, and with a quality classic item that you purchased many years ago, you will still be well-dressed today.

Talking about quality – what I said does not mean that you cannot buy quality clothing. I often purchase relatively costly items, but I do so in the hope that they will last a longer time. Unfortunately, many young men these days confuse fashion and large brand names with quality, orienting themselves by an upper-middle class ideal of consumerism. If one is looking for a role model in terms of dress style and clothing, however, it might be a better idea to take someone from the *true* upper-class as an example. Prince Charles (His Royal Highness Charles, Prince of Wales), for example, is well known and admired for his classy style. He chooses long-lived quality, and has regularly been observed wearing items he has owned for a very long time – even repaired and refurbished items. As a side note, a classic dress style also goes together better with an oldtime strongman lifestyle.

It is a sad fact that many *products of everyday use* also contain chemicals and toxins whose true effect on the body is not fully known. Especially products of artificial material are under the suspicion of being harmful, and in our days, almost everything can be produced of such materials – from cutlery, across food containers, to tools, and building material. Therefore, I try to avoid such synthetic materials, and choose traditionally designed objects of natural material wherever possible. Wood, metal, nat-

179

ural textiles, leather, stone, etc. are the materials of my choice. In many cases, these materials also have the advantage that they can be repaired when broken, which is often not the case with artificial material.

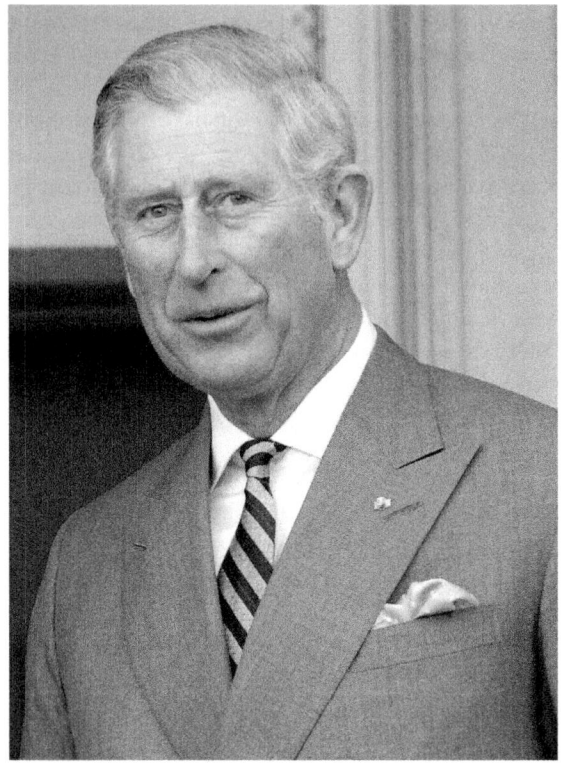

Figure 15.1 HRH Charles, Prince of Wales.

Now that I have talked about all the negative and harmful things you should avoid, let us assume a more positive and brighter outlook on life again, and consider the things you should embrace and indulge in. As hinted above, you will already know most of these as healthy and good for the body, but it can never hurt to remind us of their great importance in general, and to strength training in particular.

Getting a good night's sleep is a simple phrase, but requires awareness, discipline, and an efficient strategy. I witness again and again how many young strength enthusiasts go about their training with the best intentions, but forget all of these as soon as night falls. They waste away their nights with the senseless and excessive consumption of alcohol. Fortunately, also owing to their young age, they function well again two days later, after having passed out for a sufficient amount hours on their scanty beds. But the elements and prerequisites of a true good night's sleep, of the best sleep and most efficient rest your body can get, require careful planning throughout the day, and going rigorously against some long established customs of our society. Some examples:

- ♦ You should go to bed when you feel naturally tired, ideally when the sun sets. Preferably, this is always around the same time each day.
- ♦ You should awaken naturally, without an alarm clock, ideally when the sun rises. Preferably, this is always around the same time each day.
- ♦ You should avoid artificial light in the late evening hours, and during the night, for example when you go to the bathroom.
- ♦ Once you awaken, you should expose yourself to bright daylight soon.
- ♦ Your bedroom should be cold, dark, and quiet.
- ♦ You should not drink coffee, black tea, or other liquids containing caffeine after two o'clock PM.
- ♦ You should avoid drinking liquor in the late evenings, for example after six o'clock PM.
- ♦ You should alleviate, or divert yourself, from your worries of the day before you go to bed.
- ♦ You should get an ample amount of exercise, and clean, fresh air during the day.
- ♦ If, for whatever reason, you do not get sufficient rest during a night, you should not catch up on this lost sleep by sleeping longer in the next morning. You should go to bed earlier on the same day.

You already realize what a great effort it would be for many of us, if we actually stuck to all of these rules. However, each of us can make an effort to try to improve their sleep by paying regard to some of the items on this list. I do so rigorously whenever I can – even if it requires an amount of discipline, and saying no to some offers from people around you. I avoid coffee and black tea after two o'clock PM. Although I drink little alcohol anyway, I particularly refrain from it after six o'clock PM. I hardly ever stay late at events like festivities, celebrations, and so on. All of this may at times appear boring or anti-social, but it is a price I am willing to pay for the reward of a true good night's sleep. This being said, there are no rules without exceptions, of course.

I just mentioned the importance of exercise for your nightly sleep. Beyond your workouts, however, getting great amounts of *light natural movement*, across all joints of your body, throughout the day, is beneficial to your health in many ways. First of all, it is the obvious contrast to a sedentary lifestyle, which I already talked about above. Secondly, your body, your joints, muscles, ligaments, and bones, were designed to be in movement (at least for a large proportion of the day), rather than at rest. Children grow through movement, muscles grow through movement, and bones become strong through movement.

Now, with your oldtime strongman workouts, you will hopefully receive a sufficient amount of intense, heavy movement, necessary to build strong muscles and thick bones beyond average measures. In addition, however, you will benefit from combining this with light movement throughout the day, mainly for two reasons: 1) Light movement will keep your circulation going, ensuring your blood flow transports the necessary nutrients into your muscles for repair and growth. 2) Light movement will keep your locomotor system in shape, lubricate your joints, etc. This is, of course, a highly simplified portrayal of very complex procedures in the body. But in sum, it suffices to say that it is better for you to move a little, than to sit on a chair at a desk the whole day.

Good movements are walking, hiking, swimming, light gymnastics, and so on. Obviously, not all of my readers will have the opportunity to go swimming or hiking each day (in addition to their strongman training), especially those who make their living by working a regular job. For these, it will be best to incorporate great amounts of light movement into their regular working day.

To begin with, the best, and most natural movement for the human body is walking, as boring as it is. If you could only get one single exercise in your life, you would probably be the healthiest if you chose walking. I try to walk as much as I can during the day. Walking is a light exercise, and while taxing exercise wears you out, I firmly believe that light exercise increases your energy level (as opposed to just lying on the couch or sitting the whole day).

We all know that our bodies were not made for a sedentary lifestyle, but we have to get our (office) jobs done. Still, you could make some small changes. Take the stairs, walk to the bus station, take a walk in the midday break... I know it costs time. But perhaps it will increase your productivity so much that you get something back for it even. Do not do it because you feel you must – do it because you know that you are made for it and it is good for your body. By the way: comfortable, loose clothing helps to make movement throughout the day more fun.

While you make sure you get proper amounts of movement throughout the day in such a manner, let me add that your body also needs *periods of rest* to keep functioning well. What I mean by this is mostly one particular body part: your brain. Many of us, especially those living a sedentary lifestyle, will get ample amounts of *physical rest* throughout the day – even too much. But what worries me more is the amount of *mental rest* many of us get. Many of us hardly ever have a time during a regular working day where they are not occupied with some activity where the brain has to process input.

However, it is easier said than done to have periods of mental rest and reflection regularly. In our modern lives, there is a large, constant offer of distractions, and the temptations are great. Therefore, I suggest you plan periods of rest and reflection strictly into your daily or weekly routine. This can be, for example, in the morning, right after you get up, or during the lunch break, or in the evenings, before you go to bed. Preferably, you spend these periods alone. Social interaction is important, but requires brain activity as well. By a period of rest and reflection I mean a time that is reserved for yourself, to let your thoughts fly and do nothing else. The best example of what you can "do" in such periods is take a walk in the park or in the fields. Or you can sit in your favourite armchair with a cup of tea. I would also suggest having pen and paper ready, for any thoughts worthy of noting down that come to your head.

It seems absurd to strictly plan periods of inactivity into your weekly routine, because one might think relaxation and reflection happen by chance. However, I am a great believer in plans, routines, rituals, and structures. I am also a great believer in order. They provide security. Our modern-day lives are so busy that you will never have a problem of finding some activity to occupy yourself. The results are stress, overwhelm, and a daily routine cramped with tasks, but lacking any sense of achievement. In such a scenario it is of utmost importance to plan periods of inactivity as well. And, once you have them strictly planned (and stick to your plan whenever possible), there is a further advantage in an effect of anticipation. If your conscious and subconscious minds know that, for example, each lunch break, from Monday to Friday, is reserved for rest and reflection, you will eventually become habituated to it, automatically anticipate this break for your mind, and relax when the time comes.

There will probably be voices of people saying, "I do not have the time for periods of inactivity, because I have so much work to do." I feel with you. But if this is your subjective situation, your creativity is called upon. A period of rest and reflection can be short. Even ten minutes go a long way. You can take your break at any time during the day. It can be while you commute, on a train, or in an automobile. It can be on your working days or at the weekends only. And so on. The trick is to make it a habit, and eventually it will feel like the most natural thing to do. You should also try to get rid of the attitude that you constantly *have* to be involved in some kind of activity, even if it is only reading or communicating with friends. Your mind will benefit, and so will your oldtime strongman training.

Closely connected to such periods of rest and reflection is *peace of mind*, as the former will contribute to the latter. By peace of mind I mean that you should strive toward a state of mind where you are at peace with yourself and your surroundings. In simple words, try to become happy with how things are. By implication, if there is something about your life situation that you are not happy with, you should make an effort to either change this circumstance, or find a way to accept it. This is also one of the things easier said than done, but a serious effort of finding a creative solution or way out is better than complaining and becoming disgruntled with your life. Some situations, people, or past actions simply cannot be changed, but often there are ways around them.

Although I truly believe that peace of mind will help you with your training, I should also mention a certain paradox in connection with this. One of the great motivators for many strength enthusiasts is actually quite the opposite: A frustrating situation that causes a lot of anger can also be a great motivator, and lifting weights can be a great vent for this anger (I have hinted at this aspect above). However, while I do believe that such a motivator can result in considerable progress over a relatively long time period, I do not believe that it is desirable as a *permanent* state of mind.

As a side note, the phenomenon of frustration, anger, and similar emotions functioning as motivators for increased training intensity, are often mirrored in the kind of music that (especially young) trainees listen to during their workouts in these days. The favourite songs of these athletes typically evoke feelings of hatred, anger, frustration, aggressiveness, and so on. This must be connected to a primeval association of heavy workouts with hunting activities or waging war, i.e. atavistic human activities that *required* aggressiveness and a thirst for blood. It shall therefore be excused.

However, I have observed that constantly listening to such music during one's workouts creates a psychological *dependency*. When such trainees ever encounter a situation where they *cannot* listen to their special music (for example in a different gym), their performance and ability to concentrate drop considerably. I have conditioned myself to be immune to as many exterior factors as possible, and this includes music. I can lift heavy and set personal records to music I do not like at all, or in total silence. Personally, I prefer when no music is playing during my workouts. But when I do occasionally play music, others are often surprised by the calm and soothing music I like to listen to. This might be because I prefer to train when my mind is at peace.

I do not want to talk too much about *meaningful relationships and social interaction* here, as it is common knowledge that these factors are crucial to a fulfilled life. It is logical that they are important to have peace of mind, and thus to progress in your training. But by no means do I want to dictate how you should live your private life. First of all, this is solely your business, and, secondly, it is often not in one's hands.

This being said, I believe that in terms of organisational matters, the life of a *bachelor* is actually most suited to an oldtime strongman training and lifestyle. It is often young, unattached men who make the greatest progress in their strongman training, because they enjoy complete independence in planning workouts, purchasing and storing training equipment, and preparing meals suited to their strength endeavours. Also, if they have an income, they have free reign with their money and can decide on their own where and how they want to invest it.

Still, I do not believe that anybody will subordinate their wish of having a relationship or family to their oldtime strongman training goals, especially if they do not make their living with it. This is probably a good thing.

In terms of friends, I think any oldtime strongman will benefit from having good and close friends, especially such who are interested in the same type of training. What can be applied here in terms of an "oldtime" lifestyle is perhaps only the *number* of close friends and serious relationships one has. In our modern times it has become increasingly fashionable to have a large number of so-called friends, but rather shallow relationships with these. In fact, a meaningful relationship, even with "only" a friend, requires time, effort, and regular interaction. It is therefore not possible to have an unlimited number of good friends. It is much more rewarding to have a strictly limited number of good friends and meaningful relationships with these, which are cultivated on a regular, weekly basis.

It should be clear and self-explanatory that *clean and fresh air* and *a certain amount of sunlight* will contribute to your well-being and physical constitution. Still, there is a large amount of people who manage living almost completely without either of the two. It is a well-known fact that the proportion of people living in cities is constantly rising world-wide. Some of these cities do not even have proper parks and are highly polluted. The people living there could lead their daily lives without ever stepping out into the fresh air – if the air was fresh, that is. They leave their houses in the morning and step into an automobile, a train, or a tube. From these, they step into the building where they work. Their evenings and weekends they also spend at home. Even if they do step out of their houses to breathe the polluted air, the smog above the city keeps any sunlight from coming through.

I have mentioned earlier that the best life for an oldtime strongman is a country life – the reasons being the beneficial effect of nature on the human body and mind, the cleaner air, and the cheaper housing prices, which make it more likely to be able to afford the necessary space for a home gym. I do understand that it is not possible for everyone to live in the countryside, the reason being mostly that their place of work is in the city. In such a case, I would at least suggest you find the largest and nicest parks of this particular city, and visit them regularly. I would also suggest you make an effort and take the train at the weekends, to spend these in the countryside whenever possible.

16. The "Görner Diet"

I get frequently asked about my nutrition, probably because in the strength world, and in our modern society as a whole, there exists a popular perception that strength and muscle gains are intricately connected to strict, ascetic, and mysterious diets. I have heard claims that nutrition is responsible for a great proportion of your training efforts and results, and sometimes this proportion is said to be as high as 80 per cent. That this is nonsense is obvious. One cannot make any strength and muscle gains with a half-hearted training, even if one's nutrition is a hundred per cent perfect. The opposite, a perfect training, but without any attention to nutrition whatsoever, would probably still yield very good results.

Even if one were to consume the perfect amount and proportion of vitamins, minerals, proteins, carbohydrates, and so on, but never lift any heavy weights, he would never become stronger than average. Someone who simply eats whatever is available, but follows a rigorous workout plan, has the potential to build great strength and muscle. This is so because the body can do amazing things. It would eventually just claim the nutrients it needs from whatever tiny source it has at its disposal.

Thus, we can conclude with confidence that the most important aspect of your oldtime strongman endeavours is your *training* and not your *nutrition*. Training has the priority and nutrition comes second at best.

This being said, let me talk a little bit about my nutrition philosophy. By my use of this term, you can already see how estranged our attitude towards nutrition has become. The idea that someone even requires something like a "nutrition philosophy" reeks of decadence – considering that for thousands, even millions of years, it was humanity's primary worry to have *something* to eat in the first place. Sadly, many people in the world still find themselves in this situation from day to day. Therefore, I suggest approaching the question of the right nutrition with some humility and gratitude for the fact that so many of us *have* the option to choose what types of food we eat. It is a mere "luxury problem" that this is often such a tough choice.

Also, the thought that it can be a challenge to many people *not* to eat something (for example, sweets they want to avoid for health reasons), should strike us as an absurdity. I am grateful that I have plenty of healthy and delicious food to eat everyday. I am not picky or choosy. When invited, I hardly ever reject an offer for a meal, and my friends and family know that my heart can be won easily with a simple and hearty hot meal.

This realisation came over the years. Before it came, I tried many different diets. As a teenager, I ate any combination of protein and carbohydrates: tuna-fish with bread, cottage cheese with oranges, cottage cheese with pasta, tuna-fish with oats – you name it. For my bodybuilding competitions, I followed diets of rice, turkey, and broccoli. As a powerlifter, I would regularly lose up to 6kg (13lbs) of bodyweight within two days, prior to a competition, to be able to enter a certain weight class. I have tried low carbohydrate diets and the so-called Palaeolithic diet. (The only things I have not tried so far are vegetarianism and veganism, although I do encourage the people who follow such a diet for ethical reasons.) After having tried all of these various diets, and after coming to the realisations described above, I believe I have now found the perfect nutrition to match my oldtime strongman training: the "Görner Diet".

I have obviously named this diet after the famous German oldtime strongman Hermann Görner and his eating habits. In the classic book about this athlete, *Goerner the Mighty* (1951) by Edgar Mueller, there is a short section that describes his nutrition:

> "He is particularly partial to pork and beef and also wurst – German sausagemeat. Vegetables also, together with potatoes, but not overdoing the latter. He is very fond of nuts – particularly walnuts – and all fruits: apples especially, which he thinks every strong man should eat, as well as oranges and other citrus fruits. Cheese and eggs also figure in his diet, but he does not care for rich pastries nor does he drink milk in any quantity. As regards drinking, he drinks beer, but only moderately – seldom touches spirits..." (Mueller 112)

If we analyse this, we realize that this must have been quite a regular nutrition in Hermann Görner's days. All the foods mentioned had been available in Germany for many centuries, with the only exception, perhaps, of citrus fruit. These were probably imported from more southern European countries, like Italy or Spain. In sum, however, it was a simple, nutritious, and tasty diet, with lots of fresh and regional sources of protein, carbohydrates, fats, vitamins, and minerals: everything the body needs.

When I first read about Görner's eating habits, I was, by chance, following a Palaeolithic diet. In this diet you eat lots of vegetables, fruit, and animal protein, but avoid dairy, grain products, and starchy tubers. (I should probably mention that while I was following this diet, I had the best *looks* of my career, in terms of a low body-fat level and a satisfactory muscle tone, so I still believe that such a diet has its benefits).

When I noticed that Görner also ate little dairy products and makes no mention of bread, I asked myself whether Hermann Görner was, perhaps instinctively, following a Palaeolithic diet? If he did, he was making a big mistake, because he ate potatoes! In a strict Palaeolithic diet, you do not eat any starchy tubers whatsoever – although there are versions of this diet that allow *sweet potatoes* if the person is an athlete. At the time I read the book and was following this diet, it was very uncommon for sweet potatoes to be grown in Europe. Therefore, I would have had to buy sweet potatoes imported from regions as far away as the United States of America. You can imagine that foods coming such a long way sacrifice a large amount of their freshness, and the transporting of such foods causes unnecessary harm to the environment.

The sum of all these observations led me to the following conclusions: 1) That I should quickly do away with all this nonsense of the so-and-so-diet, and with exotic foods that are claimed to be better than regional foods. 2) That Hermann Görner simply ate basic foods that were available at his time and place – foods he enjoyed, foods that provided all the nutrients he needed to grow extremely big and strong, and foods that were healthy, because agriculture was much less harmful and aggressive at his time than it is in our days. That Görner avoided certain foods was only his personal preference. Maybe he did not tolerate them well, or he preferred other foods instead (like potatoes, rather than bread, as a source of carbohydrates).

Thus, what I mean when I talk about the Görner Diet, is not a diet in the sense of a nutrition philosophy with a marketable name that is supposed to evoke feelings of belonging to a subculture with a united morale and outlook on life. It is simply "eating what is there": basic foods, fresh, regionally sourced, traditional, and tasty. No brand names, no exotic "superfoods", no shiny packaging, nothing processed, and nothing that needs to be advertised in any way. It is actually not a diet. It is just a common sense approach to eating.

As an example, what do I eat (and what do I avoid)? Here is a simple list of the basic foods I eat about 99 per cent of the time:

- Various seasonal vegetables that grow in Austria and Germany (e.g. leek, spring onion, cauliflower, broccoli, Brussels sprouts, mushrooms, fennel, courgette, pumpkin, green beans, parsnip, radishes, peppers, cucumber, beetroot...)
- Carrots
- Lettuce
- Onions
- Garlic
- Potatoes
- Pork
- Beef
- Fish (especially trout and herring)
- Various kinds of sausage

- *Speck* (an Austrian kind of bacon)
- Eggs
- Apples
- Berries
- Bananas and citric fruit (these are the main foods I eat from time to time that are imported)
- Yoghurt
- Cheese
- *Topfen* (an Austrian kind of cottage cheese)
- Butter
- Nuts (mostly hazelnuts, walnuts, and almonds)
- Seeds (mostly sunflower seeds and linseeds)
- Olive oil
- Beans
- Oats
- Pasta
- Bread (preferably home-made)
- Vinegar
- Honey
- Herbs (mostly parsley and chive)

You will realize that this is actually quite a boring list of foods, common in the whole Western world. (If you come from a different part of the world, I am certain that there are comparable basic foods for you to choose.) Nevertheless, it is a rather long list – long enough to prepare a great variety of tasty and nutritious recipes of main dishes, various types of breakfasts, snacks, etc. These basic ingredients also have the benefit that they are relatively cheap, even if they come from quality sources (preferably directly from a farmer). Perhaps the only exceptions are meat and fish, which are, in my opinion, the two major foods where you should be willing to spend a little more money for supreme quality.

Here are my preferred drinks:

- Water
- Herbal tea (locally sourced)
- Coffee (imported)
- Black tea (imported)

Here are my preferred indulgences:

- Home-made cake
- Home-made cookies
- Home-made jam
- Chocolate (imported)
- Beer (German)
- Whiskey (Irish)

Although I can be rather ascetic when I want, I like to have homemade cake or cookies with my tea from time to time, even during periods when I try to reduce my body weight.

Another question people frequently ask me is what kinds of *supplements* I use. The short answer is, a tasteless whey protein powder, sometimes a little bit of creatine, and occasionally some vitamin C. The long answer is that the question often stems from the wrong kind of attitude. It is the perception that the use of supplements differentiates a serious strength enthusiast from a hobby sportsman: To make serious strength gains, not only a mysterious, strict, and ascetic diet is necessary, but also, sooner or later, the use of supplements. Only one who takes supplements can be considered a serious athlete, and, if one wanted to enter the club of these, one should better start taking supplements as early as possible. This is the qualifying criterion whether one is serious about his training or not – so people believe.

I honestly do not know where this nonsensical perception stems from, but it must have to do with clever marketing. People with such an attitude overlook the fact that only one who *trains seriously* is a serious strength athlete. As I said, nutrition comes second place (at best), and supplements are, as the name says, only meant to "supplement" your nutrition. They are by no means necessary. Having made clear above that proper oldtime strongman training consists of consistent, heavy workouts, and that a proper nutrition consists of basic, fresh, and traditional foods, I should not waste too much further space on supplements. I will only point out the most basic facts, *viz.*:

1. The strongmen of the old days did not use any supplements. At their time, only two different kinds of substances were consumed: food and medicine. The latter, which had the form of powder, pills, or serums, you consumed only when you were ill. To grow strong, stay healthy, and have the kind of energy to go about your daily life – especially if this consisted of hard physical labour – people considered basic, nutritious, and traditional meals the right way to go.

191

This is still perceptible in the traditional cuisine and linguistic aspects of different cultural areas. The traditional "ploughman's lunch" in Britain, for example, consists of bread, cheese, and onions. In Austria, we have a saying that if someone lacks physical strength, he has not eaten enough *Knödel* – a traditional, much cherished Austrian meal of dumplings, made from leftover breadcrumbs. In Bavaria, the rural population still believes in the strength- and energy-providing qualities of unfiltered *Weißbier* (wheat beer) – actually the type of beer with the highest amount of vitamins and minerals.

The idea that you gain muscle and strength from powders, pills, and ampoules is a rather odd and recent phenomenon. Of course, it is possible to gain strength and muscle from pills and ampoules if you take performance-enhancing drugs into consideration, but I am talking about ways to gain *natural* strength.

2. Supplements are products that can be marketed very efficiently: with brand names, shiny packagings, or celebrities as mascots. This fact in itself should advise caution. Basic foods, which provide humans with everything their bodies need since millions of years, do not require this kind of marketing. If you go to a food market to buy apples, you take a close look at them, and if they look fine, come from the right source, and the price is acceptable, you buy them. If you want to buy protein powder, you are influenced by advertising, you will have to compare the different brands, look for quality labels, look at the ingredients, and still hardly know what you are buying. It could be practically anything, coming from a questionable source, and being contaminated with all kinds of substances.

However, if you look at supplements from a business perspective, it is the ideal product to earn money with. The raw material is cheap to buy (whey, for example, is a by-product of various dairy products, and European countries already produce way too much milk. It actually has to be dried and stored in gigantic warehouses, because they literally do not know where to put it all). It is easy to create a *perceived value* to increase the profit margin (for example by putting the powder into a well-designed container, or by getting a well-known and popular strength athlete under contract to make him claim that he uses the product). Finally, because the supplement is a consumable, it can be sold to the same person over and over again. All of this you should keep in mind the next time you consider taking any kind of supplement.

3. Nevertheless, I use certain supplements (whey protein, creatine, and vitamin C), for the following reasons: A protein powder is a very cheap and practical source of protein, and it is a commonly known fact that a higher than average intake of protein (and calories in general) is necessary

for muscle growth. A protein powder can be quickly prepared and consumed, and thus generate a protein-rich meal that, if the price is fair, costs much less per one gram of protein than most other, proper protein-rich foods. I say proper, because I want you to internalize the fact that a protein powder is only a cheap and practical solution, but never one that surpasses traditional, local, and natural food sources. If I could, I would prefer a steak to a protein drink at any time.

I choose a *whey* protein powder mostly out of habit, but in fact I have considered using other protein powders as well, for example plant-based ones. There is no real good reason why an oldtime strongman should prefer a whey protein powder to any other type of protein powder to reach his goals.

I use creatine mainly for two reasons: 1) It has become a habit that I consume small amounts of creatine during periods where my primary goal is building strength (in opposition to reducing body weight). However, I really cannot tell whether my strength gains during such periods are even in part owed to this substance, or whether it has, at best, a psychological, placebo-effect. 2) I still have a package of creatine powder that is half-full as I am writing this, and I want to use it up, rather than throw it away. I do not know yet whether I will buy a new package, once this one is used up. One should also not overlook the fact that lots of foods contain creatine naturally. Herring, for example, contains relatively large amounts of this substance – in addition to protein and valuable omega-3 fatty acids.

The same rule as to protein powder applies to vitamin C: In its pure form, in which it can be purchased from any pharmacy, vitamin C is not in any way superior to that found naturally in fruit and vegetables. It is only cheap per gram, because of its concentrated form. This being said, I must give vitamin C the credit for being a wonderful essential vitamin, with all sorts of benefits. One of these is that it alleviates the processing of iron in the body, and iron is, in my eyes, one of the most important minerals for strength athletes (which makes me wonder at times why iron supplements are not advertised more than many other, much less useful substances).

Coming back to vitamin C, I consume it in powdered form because it is practical. A powder can be mixed into meals or drinks easily (obviously, only in the small doses that are recommended), if no fresh fruit are available. I always have some with me when I am touring Europe to do my strongman shows, because it saves me the hassle of finding a food market to buy fresh fruit or vegetables.

In sum, concentrated vitamin C in powdered form, although by no means necessary if you consume fresh fruit and vegetables regularly (which is always preferable), is probably the one supplement I want to condemn the least. Just consider the many lives that could have been saved if some of history's brave maritime and Arctic explorers, up to the early twentieth century, would have had concentrated vitamin C available to save them from scurvy. As a final side note, vitamin C should never be heated.

Having now explained that supplements are not really necessary, but mainly practical and cheap solutions, I want to dig a little bit deeper into the question of what the body *does* need. Above, I have claimed that a proper nutrition consists of basic, fresh, and regionally sourced foods, but it is a commonly known fact that this is not the whole story. On a more abstract level – under the microscope, so to say – the body needs certain types of *nutrients*. In the following, I will provide a simple table of the most important ones, grouped by type, and provide some examples of basic foods that contain them:

Fatty acids	Omega 3	Fish, meat, eggs, walnuts
	Omega 6	Fish, meat, eggs, walnuts
Amino acids	Histidine	Beef, fish, walnuts, eggs
	Isoleucine	Eggs, fish, beef, walnuts
	Leucine	Eggs, beef, fish, walnuts
	Lysine	Fish, beef, eggs, walnuts
	Methionine	Fish, eggs, beef, walnuts
	Phenylalanine	Eggs, walnuts, pork, Fish
	Threonine	Eggs, fish, beef, walnuts
	Tryptophan	Cacao, eggs, walnuts, pork, fish
	Valine	Eggs, fish, beef, walnuts
	Arginine	Walnuts, pork, eggs, fish
Vita-mins	A	Fish, liver, butter, eggs
	B1	Sunflower seeds, pork, liver, eggs
	B2	Liver, meat, fish, eggs, almonds
	B3	Liver, meat, fish, nuts, salad, carrots, mushrooms
	B5	Liver, eggs, nuts, fruit, vegetables
	B6	Liver, meat, vegetables, nuts, eggs
	B7	Liver, walnuts, mushrooms, fish, meat, apples
	B9	Liver, salad, beetroot, carrots, eggs, nuts, fruit
	B12	Liver, meat, fish, eggs
	C	Berries, parsley, lemon, liver, apples, onions
	D	*Sunlight*, herring, salmon, sardines, eggs, mush-rooms, liver, butter
	E	Walnuts, hazelnuts, almonds, olive oil, beetroot, salad
	K1	Cabbage, parsley
	K2	Liver, eggs, butter, beef, salmon

Minerals, trace elements	Calcium	Almonds, hazelnuts, parsley, beetroot, salt, mineral water
	Chlorine	Salt
	Potassium	Parsley, chocolate, nuts, salt
	Magnesium	Liver, fish, sunflower seeds, chocolate, berries, mineral water, salt
	Sodium	Salt
	Phosporus	Meat, fish
	Sulphur	Garlic, onions
	Iron	Liver, meat
	Iodine	Seafood
	Copper	Nuts, cacao, liver, fish, vegetables
	Manganese	Black tea, nuts, vegetables
	Molybdenum	Everywhere
	Selenium	Eggs, meat
	Zinc	Liver, meat, fish, seafood

As this table shows, all essential nutrients the human body needs can in theory be supplied by a choice of relatively simple, basic, and, one might say, boring foods. This is logical if one considers how long humans have survived on very basic diets, before the invention of fashionable nutrition philosophies, supplements, and the like. However, bear in mind that this table is only meant as an illustration, and by no means a precept of which foods you should eat and which not. It contains no information on the exact *amounts* of these nutrients a food type contains, and in some cases a balanced ratio is crucial.

With all of this knowledge, I want to wrap this section up by once more asking the simple question: What is healthy food? All sorts of groups, from scientists, across idealists, to athletes debate this question heavily. If I had the only true answer to this question, it would mean a small-scale revolution, and – unlike many other writers – I would never make such a claim. However, before I close this section, I want you to consider the following observations I have made over the years:

1. Observation: Since the beginning of humanity, humans have migrated and spread across the globe. They have since managed to survive on very different diets and in very different living conditions.

Conclusion: Humans are, in principle, very versatile and adaptable when it comes to nutrition.

2. Observation: The adaptation to different foods and living conditions often happened over long periods of time and, in some cases, lead to genetic adaptation.

Conclusion: It seems that the imagined "ideal diet" for any human individual depends on the genetic predisposition of this individual to a certain degree. As genes are being mixed through migration, in particular since the last few centuries, it is very hard to tell from the outside what the supposed "ideal nutrition" of any individual would be.

3. Observation: Nutrition experts have varying and even contradicting views on which foods can be considered "healthy" and which not. For example, some advise you to eat a strictly plant-based diet, while others advise you to eat lots of animal protein.

Conclusion: One cannot rely on one "nutrition expert" only, and must be cautious and critical with any advice pertaining to a healthy nutrition.

4. Observation: Most experts agree that fruit and vegetables are healthy in general. Nevertheless, many say that raw fruit and vegetables should be avoided in the evening hours.

Conclusion: Even within certain food groups there is a degree of relativity that can make the same food be considered healthy or unhealthy, depending on other factors.

5. Observation: In our modern world, there exist countless accusations towards large food companies, saying that they produce their food with methods that hurt our environment, cause excessive cruelty to animals, exploit workers, consume limited natural resources, and produce food of inferior quality, with possible health risks. In many cases, it is not determinable or visible whether such a company produced a certain food or not. Often, only such foods are available.

Conclusion: Nutrition involves ethical and moral issues as well.

6. Observation: There is hunger in the world.

Conclusion: Having plenty and nutritious food is no matter of course, but should inspire gratitude.

7. Observation: For the larger part of human history, humans have thrived on foods hunted and gathered in wild nature.

Conclusion: As humanity is not extinct, this form of nutrition cannot be considered unhealthy enough to disallow human survival, i.e. edible foods hunted and gathered in wild nature are in principle healthy.

8. Observation: For a considerable part of human existence, humans have thrived on animal and plant foods cultivated on relatively small farms.

Conclusion: As humanity is not extinct, this form of nutrition cannot be considered as unhealthy enough to disallow human survival, i.e. animal and plant foods from relatively small farms are in principle healthy.

9. Observation: Most ethnic groups from demarcated cultural regions have traditional foods and recipes that rest on a century-long tradition.

Conclusion: As these cultures are not extinct, their nutrition cannot be considered as unhealthy enough to disallow their survival, i.e. traditional foods and recipes that rest on a century-long tradition are in principle healthy for the ethnic groups from this specific cultural region.

10. Observation: Our planet is being polluted on a large scale with a great number of poisons, toxins, and other harmful substances – consciously and unconsciously, visibly and invisibly. Also the transportation of foods from A to B causes pollution.

Conclusion: There is no telling in advance whether a particular food, its production, or its source do not involve a specific health risk or danger to our planet.

I believe the above observations are some of the reasons why there is so much insecurity with regard to food and nutrition in our modern world. It seems that there is no such thing as the "perfect nutrition" – at best only a "less harmful" one. Any claim regarding a "perfect nutrition" must ignore the one or the other of my observations above. Everything involves a degree of relativity. Some proclaimed "healthy foods", for example, must be transported across large distances to reach its consumer, causing excessive and unnecessary pollution to our planet (the source of all our foods). Overeating, for example, is unhealthy to our digestive system, can lead to overweight, and is a waste of resources. Malnutrition, on the other hand, is unhealthy as well. And so on.

Therefore, I suggest the following solution, until we have a better knowledge of these subjects: a *middle way*. In German, we have the saying, *"Die Dosis macht das Gift,"* which roughly translates to: "The dose makes the poison." It basically means that even if the one or the other food is harmful, harm can be reduced if it is only consumed in limited quantities. Thus, go for a mix instead of an overemphasis on one particular food or an extreme nutrition style. For us, as ordinary citizens, it is impossible to investigate all of the countless aspects pertaining to nutrition in the modern world and take all of them into consideration, also because some people willingly spread false information to represent their own, often financial, interests.

If you can, avoid exotic foods that come from far away, because they cause long ways of transportation. If you can, avoid foods from large companies and choose foods from small and local farmers instead. Do not eat excessive amounts of food in general, or of one particular type of food. If you can, go for traditional foods from your region, or foods traditionally connected with your ethnic origin (mind you that not every so-called "tradition" is really a tradition). If you discover that you do not tolerate a specific type of food well, avoid it – it might have to do with your genetics and this is nothing to be ashamed of. Be critical and question origin, production method, fertilisation method, farming method, etc. of your food source. Eye nutrition extremists and gurus with suspicion.

This is, in essence, what I mean when I speak of a *proper Görner Diet*.

17. Healthcare: How I avoid having to cancel a show because of illness

Over the more than ten years that I have made money as a performing oldtime strongman, I have – voluntarily and involuntarily – come into contact with lots of artists: acrobats, musicians, jugglers, comedians, and so on. I have noticed repeatedly how almost all of them, whatever their art was, tried to take good care of their health (especially the good ones). It was obvious to me that someone who works with his body would do this, like an acrobat, but even when I ran into comedians and musicians backstage, I would catch them eating vegetables and fruit, doing yoga and gymnastics, taking a nap to catch up sleep, going for a walk in the fresh air, and so on. In short, they would do what they considered healthy for their body, based on the best of their knowledge. Hardly ever have I witnessed any of the partying, drinking, and self-destructive behaviour some would connect with the lifestyle of a "true" artist. When I once started a conversation with a comedian on this topic, telling him of my observation of how many artists try to eat and live healthy, he said (and he was not joking in this instance): "Of course. Otherwise they would not do it for long."

He had a point. If you are a performing artist, whether musician or acrobat, and especially if this is your main income, you live a special lifestyle. For example, you cannot simply stay at home when ill. When you cancel a show, there is almost always a loss of income involved – sometimes even a penalty you have to pay, because the organizer loses his show act! Have this happen to you a few times and you will surely think of some way to avoid it in future.

Likewise, the number of bad shows you can play is limited. Of course, there are many extrinsic factors that can lead to a bad performance over which you have no control. But perform badly as a comedian or musician, because you spent the night before partying and drinking, and the organizer will not book you again. Even worse, bad mouthing will cost you other bookings as well. Perform badly as an acrobat for the same reasons, and you will get hurt. It is probably not true that *all* artists live a healthy lifestyle, but those who want to enjoy long and successful careers, inevitably have to take good care of their health.

I should knock on wood, but to this day, since more than ten years, I never had to cancel a show because of illness or because of an injury. It might happen some day, as it can happen to anyone, but at least I make a serious effort to *minimize the chances* of illness and injury. I do not want to cancel a show if I can avoid it *by any means*. Compare this to the office worker with health insurance, who can take a day off when he is not feeling well, without *any negative consequence* whatsoever. In theory, it is a good thing that this is possible in our days, and we must be grateful if our country has a functioning health system. However, some people inevitably exploit this system and stay away from work, because they partied and drank the night before. This the performing artist cannot afford. He has to take over *responsibility* for his own health. Especially so when he works with his body and has to demonstrate feats that afford physical skill – be it strength, stamina, balance, coordination, speed, or flexibility.

I perform up to five 30-minute shows per day. I perform after driving 1000km (620 miles). I perform after only a few hours of sleep (not because of partying, but because of travel). At the circus, I have performed for three weeks in a row, twice a day, with no day of rest. I have performed in the gleaming Italian sun and in ice-cold Alpine winters, outdoors, topless. And each time I do, I demonstrate, and have demonstrated, feats of strength that I would challenge anyone in the audience to replicate. However stressful and troublesome my week was, when I am booked to perform on Saturday, the organizer can trust that I am there, giving my absolute best to entertain his audience. And each time I return home, driving through the night, I feel ready to do the same after a day (or two) of rest.

It is not that I am never ill. It did not happen often, but it did happen that I was dead sick on Mondays, and performing again on Friday.

What is my secret? If there is anything like a "secret" at all (there are generally not many "secrets" in oldtime strongman training), it is my attitude. This attitude has to do with taking what I do seriously and giving it a certain priority. As I said earlier, we all know what is good for our body, but most do not stick to these things too rigorously. They allow themselves a certain leeway, because they tolerate the small price they pay. During my show season, I do not take this kind of chance. I struggle every day to give my body all it needs: vegetables, sleep, periods of rest, exercise, and so on. It is a struggle, because temptations to slacken the reins are everywhere. Therefore, I consider the consequences of my actions. People party and drink at night, and block out the fact that they will feel bad the day after. People sit all day and never step out into the fresh air, knowing that eventually they will get back pain and a vitamin D deficiency. People never spend a thought on their immune system, although they know that a strong immune system protects them from a multitude of illnesses. People have the knowledge, but take the wrong actions, because they disregard the long-term consequences. But avoiding illness and feeling lousy requires long-term foresighted thinking. The actions you take today determine how you feel tomorrow, by the end of the week, next winter, or in five years. In my case, the long-term consequences would be considerable, like a loss of income when I have to cancel a show. Thus, I am forced to think long-term.

Ironically, thinking long-term requires small, day-to-day efforts, for example: making sure you get your vegetables and protein, your sleep, your exercise, your periods of rest, your meaningful social interaction, and so on, every day. Again, we all know what measures should be taken every day to stay as healthy as possible. But it seems easier said than done: go for a run twice a week, spend time with your family and friends every day, lift weights four times a week, sleep eight hours per night, eat healthy and protein-rich meals six times per day... For most of us, it is simply not humanly possible to juggle all of these aspects day after day. If we pull ourselves together, we might be able to do this for a couple of weeks, but at some point, it becomes too arduous to tell ourselves again and again, every day, to do what we are supposed to do.

From my perspective, there is only one solution to this problem. It is based on rather old-fashioned virtues: a clear weekly plan, with strict rules and a neat order. In this weekly plan, every life aspect should have its place and time: your training days and time, time outdoors, time for cardiovascular activity, time to work, time to shop, time with friends and family, even times to be wasted away with senseless activities (if you have a craving for such), as well as a strict bedtime and wake-up time (the bedtime should be more strict than the wake-up time, because ideally, you wake up when your inner clock tells you – rather than your alarm clock. Unfortunately, for most people it is the other way round: they are lenient with their bedtime and let their alarm clock wake them up).

Likewise, you should have a clear nutrition plan, not to count calories, but to make sure you get your essential nutrients on a day-to-day basis. Of course, you should allow room for some variation here, for pleasure and to avoid a one-sided nutrition. But there is nothing wrong with having some meals or snacks during the day that are always the same and consist of foods that provide essential nutrients (like the famous "apple a day").

At first sight, this strategy does not convince everyone. It is easy to formulate a plan, but the difficulty lies in sticking to it. So what you do is, you adapt this plan continuously, until it is nearly perfect and possible for you to stick to it easily. Even then, you will have to keep adapting it, as your life circumstances change. The important thing is that you have something to work with, a framework, even if this framework requires adjustments from time to time. This is quite natural. You have to experiment to find out what works for you. If your plan says, go to the gym three times per week and go for a run twice a week, but time and motivation problems keep coming up, do not blame your discipline, but adapt your plan. It is obviously not working. Go for a run only once a week and see if this works – it is better than nothing. Maybe you can increase the volume later on when you have a smaller workload, for example.

Also, it might be a good idea to combine certain life aspects. For example, make Sunday the day for a hike with your family, and combine cardiovascular activity, family time, time outdoors, sunlight, and fresh air. If you cannot sacrifice a whole day, go for a shorter hike in the afternoon. Once you seem to have a plan that works, stick to it for long enough and you will experience a phenomenon that many writers talk about (Benjamin Franklin was probably the first to mention it in his autobiography): Once you do something often and regularly enough, it will become a *habit*, and require little to no effort to stick to. The aspects I try to cover in my weekly plan, to ensure the best continuous (mental and physical) health possible, are the following:

- Time for my oldtime strongman training (of course)
- Time for cardiovascular activity
- Three main meals per day (and their preparation)
- Three snacks per day
- Time outdoors
- Time to shop for groceries
- Time for housework
- Time with close family
- Time with extended family
- Time with friends
- Time for work
- Time to read serious books
- Time to read books for entertainment
- Time for relaxation
- Time to sleep and awaken naturally (if possible)
- Time for a morning and evening routine (more on this later)

This sounds like a lot of tasks, but you will realize that they are all necessary for survival in the modern world, and to stay mentally and physically healthy! So, to combine all of this, I often have to reduce the weekly share of one aspect or the other. For example, I meet with friends only for an hour once per week. But still, this is better than nothing. If kept up continuously, it makes it possible to cultivate very valuable friendships. Likewise, if I only go for a short hike once per week, it is not much in terms of time spent outdoors and cardiovascular activity, but if done strictly *every* week, it goes a much longer way than planning to go for two huge hikes per week, but never doing it because you cannot find the time.

I hope you see what I mean. The trick is to have a time slot for each of these very important life aspects. Then, when the time slot comes, completely block out any temptation to spend the time slot for any other activity. One should try to be in the moment, realize that one can only do one thing at a time, and not worry about what other tasks will come up during that day. This can actually become a great challenge, and a fight against all sorts of odds.

As I said, formulating, and sticking to, such a plan successfully, requires a great amount of experimenting, experience, self-awareness, and heeding of your body's signals. All of these skills or aspects are generally important to maintain physical and mental health, regardless of your weekly plan. They have helped me a lot in to avoid having to cancel a show because of illness or injury.

It has happened even to me that despite the measures I take each week, I happen to feel ill or in pain. But what I do then, even at the slightest signal of illness or pain, is I take immediate action and formulate a plan. My aim is then to get back on track as fast as possible, for example through reducing my physical activity, through increasing my periods of rest, through stretching or recovery exercises, and so on. Once I *am* back on track, I live as wild as ever, and challenge (and thus train), my body and immune system. I do so with heavy workouts, spending time outdoors (regardless of the weather), taking ice baths, walking barefoot, and so on.

It is a question of attitude to take care of yourself. When I once asked my mentor whether he thought tiger balm would help against joint pain, he said:

> "Yes, but not because of the tiger balm. The Chinese say tiger balm only helps to scare away flies. But it helps if you treat your joints with tiger balm, simply because you do something, because you take an action, rather than doing nothing. You are telling yourself that you are taking care of your body. And this kind of attitude helps."

By now, I luckily know many of the health issues I typically have, and I know what I can do in such a case and what really works. For example, when I feel pain in my back and hips, I question whether I have been sitting too much lately. Then I try to walk more during the day and do stretching exercises for the hip extensors. If I fall seriously ill, it might even be necessary to take medication for a short while. One should not ignore the advancements of modern medicine and pharmacy and be grateful for them (despite all the harm that these industries continue to cause). But, just to make sure, I see medication as a short-term, emergency measure and refrain from it as soon as I recover.

All of this comes with experience, and I am still learning. But the important aspect is to become habituated to listening to your body's signals, to take them seriously, to try to interpret them, and to take action accordingly – be it recovery exercises, changing one's lifestyle, stretching, or asking a colleague for advice. It might even involve seeing a doctor or taking medication as a last resort. At the end of the day, however, as I have tried to show, my profession as an oldtime strongman forces me work to hard to *prevent* any kind of illness or medical condition wherever that lies in my power. Just imagine how much it would relieve a country's social security system if all people would think and act this way (and how much less doctors and pharmacy companies would earn).

18. Morning and evening routines and their benefits

In the preceding chapter I already hinted at the fact that a morning and an evening routine are integral parts of my weekly schedule. To introduce such into my daily routine is an idea I have long had in the back of my mind. However, it was an article by Brett and Kate McKay, on the morning routine of the oldtime strongman Adrian Peter Schmidt, that eventually inspired me to develop my individual morning workout routine and stick to it. I have done so ever since.

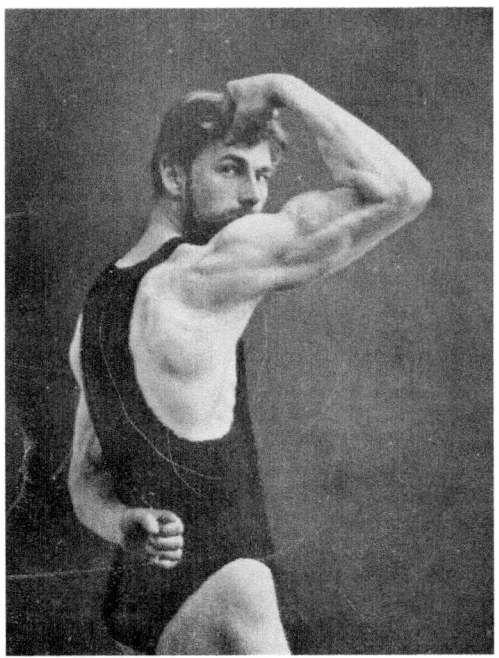

Figure 18.1 Adrian Peter Schmidt.

My morning workout routine is similar to the one recommended by Schmidt, but it differs in several respects. The ideas behind it are the following: A *very* short and *very* light exercise routine, done *every day*, sometime between getting out of bed and breakfast, and which can be done anywhere. In my case, it consists of several exercises – part gymnastics, part dynamic stretching – that mimic all of the basic human movement patterns described above (walking/running/jumping, throwing, lifting, climbing, dexterity, hitting, biting). I could describe the exercises here, but they are very basic, and I recommend you simply come up with your own choice of exercises that suit you. I only do very few repetitions per exercise, and the routine is so minimalistic that it takes three minutes at the most. It is easy and not exhausting at all.

Despite – or because of – these limitations, it has, among others, the following benefits:

- ♦ I never skip it (because the effort is so minimal).
- ♦ It activates all the major muscles, bones, ligaments, tendons, and joints in your body, at the start of every day.
- ♦ It wakes up your nervous and circulatory system, and makes you feel alive and fresh, before breakfast.
- ♦ This being said, you never breakfast without at least *any* preceding exercise.
- ♦ It allows you to quickly check how you feel on a given day, whether you experience stiffness or pain in any movement or any part of your body.
- ♦ You have a short mobility session every day.
- ♦ It can be done on days with a low energy level as well.
- ♦ It makes you feel manly and old-fashioned.

You will agree that these are quite a few benefits for only three minutes per day. They are the reasons why I have never stopped doing a daily morning routine ever since I took up this habit. It is an integral part of my mornings that I never ever leave out, just like brushing my teeth. Hopefully, you will discover a morning routine that works for you and experience some of these benefits as well.

I also have a corresponding evening routine. However, I do not perform it *every* day, simply because I feel too tired sometimes. But when I do it, any time between finishing my daily chores and brushing my teeth, it is a very slow, thoughtful stretching routine, not unlike what some people would call yoga, or, more specifically, the so-called "Sun Salutation" (although I do it in the evenings). It is not as fast and "active" as the morning routine, because it is meant as a ritual to bring the day to an end and prepare myself for sleep. It is designed to stretch all the important muscles in the body that tend to shorten, for example after long hours of seated activity, like office work or driving. It only takes three minutes as well (although it could be repeated as often as one liked) and feels fantastic.

It has the following benefits:

- It is a ritual that helps to slow down and shut down your system after a hard day.
- It increases mobility in all the important joints.
- It stretches the muscles that tend towards shortening.
- It relaxes your muscles and locomotor system before sleep, to avoid stiffness in the morning.
- It gives you three minutes at the end of the day to relax your mind as well.

Perhaps you will find an evening routine that works for you and does not require a great effort, so that you stick to it. I do not believe that an evening routine is as essential as a morning routine, but if you find the daily motivation, it helps your body and mind tremendously. If you are religious, you can combine it with some sort of prayer, meditation, or saying grace.

19. Performing: How to perform feats of strength in front of an audience and how to develop a show. With a few pieces of advice on such performances, and a comment on mental strength.

While I am not the absolutely strongest man on earth, and while there are lots of men alive who are way stronger than I in one way or another – naturally or with the help of forbidden substances – I think I can safely say that there are not many who have the sort of *natural all-round strength* combined with *longstanding stage experience* that I call my own. By stage experience I do not simply mean stepping on a lifting platform and lifting a weight in front of a crowd. I mean stepping in front of an audience, entertaining and inspiring them for a considerable amount of time (through the demonstration of old-fashioned feats of strength), completely on my own, and in such a professional and organized manner that it is theoretically possible to make a living of it.

I am not trying to show off with this experience, as it was, to a large degree, luck, and the doing of other persons that made me end up with this opportunity. But I hope that I will be able to *pass on* to others some of the knowledge I have acquired in this way, and I hope that some will make good use of it. In particular, I hope that this information will not only be helpful to people who want to do the exact same thing as I (i.e. doing oldtime strongman shows for a living), but also for anyone else, and for many different situations in their lives.

By the way, if you do plan to become a performing oldtime strongman, or if you already are one, and if this information I am about to give you will be of any help whatsoever, I hope you will write to me and let me know of your successes. I also hope you will give me some credit, like mentioning me in your memoirs you will write some day.

How a demonstration of feats of strength should be designed, and whether it will be successful or not, depends heavily on the context, and, inextricably connected to this, the audience. Feats of strength can be demonstrated in all sorts of contexts: in circuses, in variety shows, on the street (for "hat money" or through a paid booking for a street festival), at historical fairs, at company celebrations, at sporting events, for an advertising campaign, at charity events, in schools and kindergartens, in a private context (like birthday parties or weddings, whether for money or for friends), in informal contexts (like in a pub), and so on.

I have done all of this, and I can tell you that depending on the context, a strength demonstration becomes a totally different task – with different requirements, different degrees of difficulty, and different chances of success. Compare, for example, the context of a circus to the context of a street festival. In the circus, your show is supposed to be short, sensational, and only accompanied by music – you are not supposed to talk. At a street festival, you are supposed to do nothing but talk and stretch your show out to become lengthy. It is no problem on the street to show mediocre, but entertaining feats.

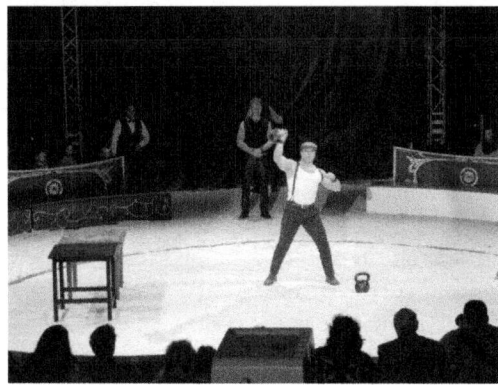

Figure 19.1 Performing in the circus.

Or, compare the context of a weightlifting event to that of a school carnival. In front of weightlifters you will have to demonstrate much more challenging and exotic feats of strength to impress anyone, whereas pupils will be thankful for any change to their day-to-day school life whatsoever. However, school children, if you do not manage to inspire their sympathy, will sabotage you mercilessly, whereas grown up weightlifters will usually treat you with some courtesy, even if they think your show is lousy.

Unfortunately, I do not have the space here to go through all these different contexts and the different challenges they provide. However, from my experience, if you have the opportunity to choose, a family audience is always best. It is a mixed audience, with grown ups and children of different ages, and women and men. If you do not please one part of this audience, maybe you will please another. Also, parents will usually look after their children to a certain degree, and admonish them if they try to sabotage you (although there are also the sorts of parents who do not care), and they will be thankful for the entertainment and inspiration you offer their children. Mind you, however, that there will always be some fathers who will feel uncomfortable at the idea of their children seeing someone stronger than themselves.

Whatever the context is, there are some techniques to make your show more effective. By effective I mean achieving certain aims. As you are there to perform, or demonstrate, something, one aim should be to demonstrate it to *as many people as possible* – otherwise you could do it only for yourself, in a locked room at your home, as well. Thus, you need to *attract and keep* your audience's attention – whoever the audience is. Secondly, you want your feats of strength to succeed. You do not want to announce, "Now I will bend this big spike!" and then fail to do so. This is the nightmare of any performing strongman, and you would not believe how often I still dream of such a scenario at night (although I have never failed at any feat in any of my shows). Thirdly, the purpose of a strength demonstration is to demonstrate *superior* strength – it would be meaningless to perform a feat that anyone in the audience could replicate. Thus, you have to make sure nobody in the audience can do what you do, and will potentially embarrass you. Fourthly, you want your audience to be well entertained. In the best case, you want them to be excited, amazed, laugh, cry, or whatever – in short, inspire an emotion in them. But at least you do not want to bore them.

Let me now go through a few pieces of advice on how to increase your chances to achieve all of this. The first aspect I want to talk about is costume, and I call it costume on purpose, because this is how you should perceive your outfit on the day of your demonstration. As a performer, you are supposed to grab the attention of the audience, make yourself the centre of attention, and stand out from the crowd. The easiest way to do this before you even start your show, is to attract attention through your outward appearance. If there is something about your appearance that makes people turn their heads while you approach your show spot, you have already won the first fight. You outward appearance should signal: "Here I am, I am someone special, and I have something special to show to you – look at me." I do not mean that this has to be in a flamboyant or obnoxious way. It can be as simple as wearing a suit where everybody else is dressed in sporting clothes. But your costume should obviously fit the context, and as there are countless possible contexts, there are no further general rules regarding costume. I could say it should be clean and neat, but even this is not generally true, because at medieval festivals I often wear a dirty and torn shirt on purpose, to provide a feeling of nostalgia and authenticity.

By the way, what can be said of your costume can also be said of your props. They should look interesting and fit the context. This is why I have stopped rolling up modern frying pans at historical festivals, for example. But more on the choice of props later.

First, I want to talk about how to attract and keep the attention of a crowd. This is not necessary in every context, as in a circus, but in many others it is crucial, for example on the street. For many, it is an unpleasant thought to make themselves the centre of attention, but if you want to demonstrate something to a crowd, there is no way around it.

Common ways to attract attention are acoustic means, visual means, humour, and suspense. Music, for example, is a great acoustic means to attract attention, and most successful street artists simply start by playing loud and interesting music, or an exotic musical instrument, which automatically draws people towards the source. Another way to attract attention acoustically would be with your voice, especially when it is amplified in some way. It is a less pleasant way than music, as loud speaking can be a nuisance and even drive some people away from you. Whether it works or not, depends heavily on the context. In some contexts, people will flock towards you even if you insult them (in a playful way), in other contexts, people will shun you even if you are extremely nice and friendly. Experimenting and experience go a long way here.

Visual means to attract an audience are, besides your costume, interesting *props* and *height*. If you stand on an elevation, like a stage, a chair, or any other large construction, people will automatically look at you. Regarding props, take a clown, for example. A good clown will usually have a huge suitcase or box full of unusual and funny items. The unloading of such a suitcase in itself can already attract an audience's attention.

Here we are already bordering humour and suspense. If the clown's props are funny, or if he does funny things with them, playfully and casually, the people who are already there will laugh and want for more. The laughs of these people will attract the attention of others. Also, there might be some interesting props he does not interact with yet. These will create suspense in the audience, who wonders, "What is this thing for?" They will stay to find out. This can also be done in a straightforward and obvious manner. The performer might tell the audience, "By the end of this show, I will demonstrate what this thing is for!" or, "By the end of this show, I will do this or that with this thing." This is like a silent contract with the audience to stay until the end.

There are some further means to heighten the chances that people will stay until the end (if it is a context where they can, theoretically, leave during the show). First of all, duration: If the show gets too long, chances increase that people will start having a hard time to concentrate, and leave. Good street artists can hold an audience for up to 45 minutes, and keep their show interesting and entertaining until the very end. But, as a rule of thumb, the human attention span lies somewhere between 15 and 20 minutes. Thus, as a beginner, your show should ideally be somewhere within this range. Even so, however long your show will last, it might be a good idea to tell your audience in advance. If they know what to anticipate, they will automatically set their inner clock to this duration. This inner clock works amazingly well. For example, when you say in the beginning that your show will last thirty minutes, but surpass this mark, people will slowly get nervous after almost exactly thirty minutes, become restless, and the first ones will start to leave.

Next, it helps to have a well-rounded show with effective transitions from one feat to the next, with a clear flow, and without interruptions. I guess that ideally, your show has something like a story line, where one part leads directly to the next – although I have never used this concept so far. Be aware that a simple row of feats of strength, not connected to each other in any way, are like a series of mini-shows, giving anyone in the audience the opportunity to leave after each feat.

Much of the success of your show also depends on your communication with the audience. Here, endless skills come into play, and I cannot go into detail with all of them. One could acquire and utilize techniques derived from such diverse fields as rhetoric, acting, storytelling, breathing, theatre, dancing, etc. for a live strongman performance. One easy way to not worry too much about such skills would be to work with an assistant – a bottler, or barker, or however you want to call it – someone who presents and introduces you as the strongman, like a circus director or a market crier at a funfair. This person does all the communication with the audience for you, while you remain mostly silent. This method is traditionally associated with the strongman, more so than with other genres of the performing arts. Among the reasons for this are the potential dangers and risks that accompany a demonstration of strength, including envy from someone in the audience and consequential attempts of sabotage. Thus, the assistant also has the function of having the strongman's back. Another reason for the frequent use of an assistant in the strongman genre is that strength athletes do often not belong to the communicative type.

If you do not want to, or cannot, work with an assistant, you will have to do all the communication with the audience yourself. As I cannot go into detail here, I want to condense all the important aspects into one principal aim you should have: to try to project as much *confidence* as you can. This is done, in the first place, by *being* confident (which is easier said than done). However, it *shows* in your voice and body language. For example, if your voice is low in volume, high in pitch, fast in pace, and consists mostly of mumbling, and if you repeatedly run out of air, your audience will automatically associate this with insecurity and a lack of self-confidence. In terms of body language, the same is true if you interlock your arms and hands, if you hide behind props, fidget nervously, or avoid eye contact. Thus, avoid these kinds of things. Also, try not to turn your back on your audience. Keep you hands free when you speak, use them to gesticulate, speak slowly, loudly, and clearly, stand erect, turn towards your audience and look them in the eye. This does not mean that you need to be arrogant. It is better to remain humble and friendly – but confident.

The next question is *which* feats of strength are suitable for a performance. First and foremost, you should only perform feats that fulfil at least two basic criteria:

1. You must be absolutely confident that you master the feats, i.e. that you succeed in them any time you try, even when you have a bad day. Otherwise, if your show consists of feats you can only do on a *good* day, and your day of performance happens to be a *bad* day, you have no show. Here, much depends on the type of athlete you are. There are those who perform best when under pressure. The adrenaline of being watched by a large audience will boost their performance. Then there are those who are strongest in training, in familiar surroundings. They tend to fail under pressure, e.g. when being watched. Obviously, if you want to do a strongman performance, it helps if you belong to the first type.

2. As I already mentioned, you must be confident that nobody in the audience can duplicate the feat easily, or at least no regularly strong man from the street. This is so for obvious reasons. What gives you the right to give a strongman performance and call yourself a strongman, if there are several people in the audience who can do the same?

Apart from these there are more aspects to consider when selecting your feats. Every successful feat of strength has something that I call a "script": an image it creates, or an impression it makes. The script is like a simplified description without details, like the essence of the feat. It is how an amateur who witnesses a strongman performance would narrate the feat, for example: "Yesterday I was at a circus and there was a strongman. He lifted 18 people at once!"

The script is like a "message" that the feat of strength contains, which should reach the audience and remain with the audience. It is delivered via specific "means of communication". The means of communication are the details, like the tools, technique, and secrets of the strongman, and they are not part of the script. For example: "The strongman lifted 18 people with the back lift technique. He used a self-made platform constructed of steel. The weight of the 18 people totalled 1,200kg (2649lbs) and he lifted it exactly 8.5cm (3.3in). He wore very flat shoes with rubber soles to avoid slipping. With six months of training, any reasonably strong man could do the same." These are the facts that an expert might be interested in, or an envier who wants to demystify the feat of strength, destroy the illusion, and deconstruct the script. It is not unlike a magical trick that has a script like, "The magician pulled a rabbit out of his hat."

This is the take-home message, so to say. But it should not be relevant to the audience where the magician purchased the hat, whether it had a false bottom, what breed of rabbit it was, and, most of all, how the magic trick worked.

This is how an aspiring strongman should approach a feat of strength. The clearer, simpler, and more general the script is, the better. Ideally, it can be expressed with very few words, is understandable to everyone, requires no specialized language, and has few adjectives. This is why feats of strength work best with everyday objects. The script is what the oldtime strongman should focus on when he wants to demonstrate the feat of strength to a layman or a general audience. In contrast to the script, the "means of communication" can be endlessly complex, but they should not concern a general audience – only the strongman himself and an expert audience.

Here is an example for a successful script of a feat of strength seen in a variation of the Cirque du Soleil production *Alegría*:

> "There was a strongman who lifted a weight with his teeth that two men from the audience could not lift off the floor together, and with their hands!"

The "means of communication" were, among others:

> "The weight was a round metal bar loaded with ten kettlebells. The bar had a very thick diameter. The 'volunteers' were instructed in detail by an authority, a circus clown, on how to attempt to lift the weight. The clown had also selected the volunteers. He ordered them to use a double overhand grip on the bar and lift with the strength of their legs, i.e. to start from a very low squatting position (to reduce the strain on their backs, so to say). Reportedly, the strongman Stepan Ivanov, who did the feat, can lift more than 400kg (883lbs) in this manner, so the kettlebells might have weighed up to 40kg (88lbs). But even so, let us assume they were lighter and only weighed 24kg (53lbs) each. By ten, this equals 240kg (530lbs). Two men tried to lift this. Only men with a very strong grip could deadlift half of the load, 120kg (265lbs), off the floor with a double overhand grip on such a thick bar. After the attempt of the volunteers, the strongman attached a long chain to two places on the bar, with a mouthpiece on its centre. He straddled the bar, put the mouthpiece in his mouth, and lifted the weight with mouth and hands on the chain simultaneously. He lifted it only a few centimetres off the floor. When he

stood straight, he let go with his hands. For a few seconds, he supported the weight with his teeth only, while the chain rested against his chest and took some of the load away from his teeth."

As you can see, the "means of communication" are not the business of the amateur audience, as such a close analysis can ruin the script. Also, note that the difference between "script" and "means of communication" does not equal cheating. Supporting even 240kg (530lbs) with the teeth in such a manner is a tremendous achievement. And, perhaps, it was even heavier than this and weighed 400kg (883lbs)?

Once you have made your choice of feat, you have different options of presenting it. Let us assume you want to bend a horseshoe in front of an audience to demonstrate your strength. I will give you two examples of how this could be done, and of the communication with the audience. First example:

You take a horseshoe out of your bag.
You: "This is a horseshoe. I will now bend it."
You take your wraps out of your bag and carefully wrap the horseshoe. You get ready to bend it and take a few deep breaths. You bend the horseshoe, unwrap it, and show it to the audience.
You: "Now I have bent it."
People applaud. You go on to the next feat of strength.

This is one possibility. Here is another one:

You grab your bag.
You: "All right, ladies and gentlemen, here I have an interesting object for you. Does anyone know what this is?"
You pull out the horseshoe and show it to the audience.
Children in the audience: "A horseshoe!"
You: "That's right! Now, what do you think I will do with it?"
Children: "Bend it!"
You: "Exactly!"
You pull out the wraps and wrap the horseshoe while you continue to speak.
You: "And let me tell you: There are only few people in the world who can bend a horseshoe like this. It will not be easy, because I feel a little tired today, but I will try my best – just for you."
You get ready to bend it and give it a first try, but nothing happens. Some children in the audience laugh.
You: "Hey, this is pretty tough. Have some patience, ladies and gentlemen. By the way..."

You start scanning the audience with your eyes.
You: "Does anyone of you want to have a go first?!"
Some children raise their hands.
You: "Thank you my friends, but I was always told to pick someone my size."
You approach a grown man in the audience.
You: "How about this gentleman right here? Sir, could you do me a favour? Could you testify that this is a real horseshoe and that it is pretty tough to bend?"
Hopefully, the man is a good sport, steps on the stage and gives it a try. Nothing happens. You: "Sir, can you confirm that this is a real horseshoe, that it is not made of rubber, and that it is tough to bend?"
Hopefully, the man confirms.
Man: "Yes it is!"
You: "Thank you very much, sir. Ladies and gentlemen, would you give this brave gentleman a round of applause for testifying, please!"
The man leaves the stage.
You: "All right. I must admit, until now I have not really tried. But I will now. Just give me a second."
You take a few deep breaths.
You: "Ladies and gentlemen! Are you ready!?"
Crowd: "Yes!"
You: "One! Two! Three! Go!"
You bend the horseshoe half way. The crowd applauds.
You: "Almost half-way through! This is tougher than I thought. Once more. Can you give me some support?"
The audience cheers you on, as you finish the bend. You unwrap the horseshoe and proudly present the bent shoe.
You: "There you go, ladies and gentlemen! Thank you very much!"
The audience applauds some more.

These are examples, but I hope you see the difference. In both examples, the feat itself is the same – the same horseshoe, the same technique, and the same result. The first example is a pure demonstration, which is totally fine, and in some contexts perhaps the right way to go. The second example, however, is something completely different. It is a *show*. With very little extra effort, the strongman communicates directly with the audience, involves them, answers to their needs (giving them the information they need to appreciate the feat). In short, he focuses on the audience, rather than only on himself. He creates suspense, making it unsure whether he will succeed. He demands their support, giving them the feeling they can help him finish the feat (and if they help him, they will automatically like him, because, by reverse psychology, they will subconsciously think that they would not help somebody they did not like).

Also, you should always give (someone from) the audience the possibility to check the authenticity of the feat, i.e. check your props, weigh them in their hands, etc. It is one of the downsides of the strongman genre that there is no telling from afar how difficult some feats of strength are. Even so, if an amateur from the audience checks your horseshoe, for example, it is impossible for him to tell whether it is only *pretty tough* to bend, or whether it requires *world-class strength*.

Thus, I believe the show aspect in an oldtime strongman performance is all the more important in our modern times. People will not necessarily care whether the feat is world-class or not, but they want to experience the excitement, the suspense, the physical effort, the flexing muscles, and the feeling of relief when you succeeded. And, quite often, they also want to laugh. Therefore, I hope you will agree that in many contexts, the second example would be the better way to present a feat of strength (although it is not even particularly ingenious, funny, or sophisticated). To present a feat of strength in an original way, your creativity is called upon.

The athlete in the second example above also utilizes a special technique that helps many performing artists to present their feats with more effect, i.e. to make them more suspenseful and demanding in the perception of the audience. I am talking about a three-act (narrative) structure. In storytelling, and in particular in the medium film, the three-act structure is the simplest way to tell a story. An act, or rather the ending of an act, equals a change in the basic quality of a situation, which can either be positive or negative. These basic qualities alternate. For example, you have the story of a medieval knight, who does lots of heroic deeds. Thus ends the first act – positive. Then, in the second act, lots of troubles stand in the knight's way. His damsel is caught by an evil fairy and incarcerated in a castle, protected by a dragon. By the end of this second act, the knight seems in a hopeless situation – negative. Finally, the knight overcomes these odds, slays the dragon, and frees the damsel in distress. End of third and last act: Everything has turned to good – positive. If one wanted to transfer this to a live performance in the circus arts, the difference between positive and negative would obviously be between succeeding in a feat or not.

A little anecdote as an example: When I worked in a circus a couple of years ago, the show program included a magnificent tightrope walker. On the day of the premiere, I watched his performance through the curtain and was impressed. Everything in his show was perfect and to the point– a real professional. Then, after a couple of minutes of his show, the circus director would announce the grand finale: a double back flip on the rope! Drum role. Lights on the artist. The audience fell silent. The man closed his eyes and took a few deep breaths. Then he opened his eyes again and went out onto the rope, carefully and in deep concentration. He built up momentum, jumped... and missed the rope and landed on the mat on the floor below. A wave of disappointment went through the crowd. The artist got to his feet, looked at the ground and shook his head. But then, after a few seconds, something clicked in his head. He straightened, looked up, and scanned the audience. He raised his arms and began clapping his hands with large, slow movements. He invited the audience to do the same. In a slow rhythm, the whole audience clapped their hands. He signalled to the circus director: He would try again! He got back on the platform, took a few deep breaths again, went out on the rope, built up momentum, jumped... and did it! He landed on the rope after a double back flip! The crowd went crazy. The act was over.

What had been the problem in his first attempt? Had he been nervous, because it was the premiere? I watched his show a couple of times after this and guess what? Each and every time he tried to do the double back flip the first time, he failed! And each and every time he tried it the second time he succeeded! And each and every time, the crowd went crazy. It was all show. It was a deliberate three-act structure to heighten the suspense and it worked.

The same can be done in a strongman performance. However, it is important not to overdo it. Ideally, for the greatest effect, you use this technique only once: for your grand finale, for your last (and most difficult) feat – after you have already demonstrated that you are incredibly strong. It will make your final feat appear even more difficult, it will heighten the suspense, and it will create a great feeling of relief and joy in your audience when you finally *do* succeed.

With this, I have already touched upon the question of how a strongman performance should be structured. Most of this applies only if your demonstration consists of *several* feats of strength, and not a single feat, like some record attempt (for example towing a large truck with your teeth). So let us assume you have chosen a couple of feats of strength you want to demonstrate. There are not many rules as to how they should be stringed together to result in a show. However, I have already hinted at one general rule: Your greatest feat of strength should be the final one, so that you can close your show with an impressive finale.

Mind you that "greatest" feat does not necessarily mean "most difficult" feat, but rather "most impressive to the audience". This can mean that you might have to *sell* it as the most difficult feat. For example, even if you trained hard to tear a deck of cards, and even if this is really the most difficult feat to you, it is not a good choice for the finale, because the prop is very small. However, if you have a feat of strength that is rather easy for you, but involves a large prop, and a volunteer from the audience, like pressing some sort of "human dumbbell" overhead, this might be a great choice for your final feat. The props are large, it involves height, it appears risky, and everyone can estimate how difficult it is.

The next rule is to *start* your show with a similarly impressive and large feat (but not as grand as your finale). This is so for obvious reasons: In many contexts, you want to attract the attention of your audience (or gather more people) at the beginning. Thus, you should have a strong opener that demonstrates immediately that you have something to show for, that you are not an impostor, and that you will guarantee a good show. Once you have all eyes on you, you can continue with a mediocre feat of strength, or a smaller prop, like a deck of cards. In many different genres, from theatre to music, good and successful performances have a strong opener.

Once you have selected your feats of strength, started with a good opener, shown several solid feats of strength, and closed with a real highlight, what next? Do you simply bow and walk off the stage? Of course, it depends on the context. In a circus you would, and in a variety show probably as well. However, if it is any kind of demonstration that involves direct communication with the audience, you should somehow wrap up your show. For example, thank your audience and give them a final take-home message. If it were a street performance, this would be the moment to collect hat money. This collecting of money, or "bottling", is a science in itself, and I do not want to go into detail with it here, as there is lots of information available by expert street artists who have much more skill and experience in this interesting field than I.

However, I want to talk a little bit more about an aspect I have broached several times now: interaction with the audience. As I said, interaction with the audience can help a lot to attract attention and to make your show more interesting to watch. In some cases, it can also be a necessity, because you might need assistance from volunteers from the audience (for example, to verify the authenticity of a certain feat, or to serve as a human weight).

I should also mention that especially as a performing strongman, interaction with the audience could become a very important issue. Strongmen are exposed to a greater risk of sabotage than other performing artists. Before I scare you too much, I should say that most people in an audience are, by a general rule, benevolent. They have an inbuilt barrier to wilfully displaying evil-mindedness in front of a large audience. It is only a small percentage of the general population who do not have this barrier by nature. Also, children still have to build this barrier and hone it by education. Finally, some drunkards lose it temporarily in a state of intoxication.

If one of these is the case, and if these people have made bad experiences in their lives and carry a grudge, they will look for situations to let this grudge out on other people with the largest possible damage they can cause (and still get away with). It can also be children, and, if charismatic enough, they will captivate other children to turn them against you. In such a way, one wrong person in the audience can ruin a whole show. This has happened to me several times, and I should say that there is no sure-fire method against it if the person is dedicated enough. Also, you cannot count on the civic courage of your audience. Instead of interfering and trying to help you, they will probably just watch what happens next. But do not be discouraged. First, this is the exception. Second, there are some general rules and techniques to avoid such a situation, or at least to better it.

First of all, let us look at the question why strongmen are more likely to be sabotaged than other artists. Well, first of all, by stepping in front of an audience and proclaiming that you are a strong man, you automatically imply that you are *stronger* than your audience. As muscle mass and strength are defining secondary sex characteristics, they can, on a certain level, be equalized with defining aspects of *being a man*. Thus, you imply that you are manlier than any man in the audience. You already realize the great potential for conflict in this. Secondly, it is a defining aspect of the oldtime strongman genre to demonstrate feats of maximum strength, which is a very basic skill. You do not typically demonstrate feats of agility, like an acrobat, or of coordination, like a juggler, or a combination of such with maximum strength (although there are such feats of strength). While everyone admires a great highwire walker, there are not many men in the audience who envy him, because he says, implicitly, "Look at me, I have unusual balancing skills, but I also take a great risk you would not want to take." Opposed to this, the strongman says, "Look, I can lift this weight, but you cannot, because you are too weak." This infuriates some men in the audience instinctively.

However, as long as you remain a strongman, you will not be able to change this basic premise. It lies in the nature of your art. One way to go would be to appear so frightening and dangerous that people will simply not dare to attack and sabotage you, even if they wanted to. This might work for a strongman of the "giant" type, in particular if he has a qualified assistant. Another way, and in our times probably the better way, would be to try to inspire sympathy in your audience, so that they *want* you to succeed, rather than to fail. As tastes differ, there is no sure-fire method that guarantees you will win the heart of everyone. A person liked by many will always be hated by others. However, I believe it can never hurt to be polite to your audience, be friendly to the children, and, at the same time, be confident without being arrogant. Have eye contact with your audience. This will signal confidence and make them feel directly addressed. Also, build some humour and self-irony into your show. In addition to this, one should not offend anyone in the audience in a blatant way, insult volunteers, say offensive things, or use curse words.

While I am at it, let me say a few things about how you should incorporate volunteers from the audience into your show. This involves two challenges (besides the risk that a volunteer will knowingly try to ruin your show, which I will cover later): 1) getting a suitable person to assist you in the first place, and 2) making sure that they do not feel bad about it (which already lowers the risk that they will try to sabotage you).

As to 1), there are different strategies of finding a volunteer. By the way, I call them volunteers, although they often might not help you voluntarily, because you will have to choose someone and persuade them to assist. Which of these is more suitable depends on the feat and the situation. For example, if you want to use a lady from the audience as a human weight, it might be better to *choose* someone. Otherwise, it might happen that a too weighty lady steps forward and you will have to send her back, thereby hurting her feelings. If you need a child to assist you, it might be better to ask for a true volunteer. Firstly, because children are more likely to volunteer anyway, and secondly, because you should never force a child to do something it does not want to do.

Now, let us assume you need to choose someone from the audience to assist you, someone who would not step forward of their own accord. A good clown will have the sort of charisma and authority that makes it impossible for anyone in the audience to reject a request of assistance. Also, he will simply pull someone forward, without even asking, and the person will not feel too bad about it (again, if he is a *good* clown). You can try the same if you have the corresponding authority and skill, but I do not think it is the best way to go for an athlete. I believe a strongman should project a different image than a clown. Hence, an alternative would be a more friendly, polite, and open way. For example:

Announce that you will need an assistant for the next feat, and scan the crowd with your eyes. You will notice that some people maintain eye contact with you, while others avoid it. Those who maintain eye contact are the ones who mind assisting you less. Silently make a choice of a suitable person and one or two alternatives. Approach your first choice, look them in the eye, smile, and ask very politely if they mind helping you for a minute. Give them the feeling that you do not have any evil plans with them. If they hesitate even for a second, you can be persistent, but quite frank and honest, and *say* that you do not have any evil plans: "Do not worry, you will not get hurt and I will not make a fool of you." Do not let them hesitate for too long, because once the idea gets in their heads that they have the *option* to decline, they might stick with this option. This can also become a problem when your first choice declines and there is nothing you can do to make them change their mind. This increases the risk that your second and third choice will also decline, because they see that there is this option.

As you can see, with this method you run a much higher risk of not finding any suitable candidate. Nevertheless, I think for a strongman it is better not to provoke, and not force anyone in the audience. If someone does not want to assist you at all, then so be it. This is especially true if it is a lady. It might be, for example, that she is pregnant and worried about her child, but does not openly want to reveal this fact. Now, if you stay persistent and ask again and again, for example, "Why? Why do you not want to help me? Come on!" you will put her in a very compromising situation.

There are, of course, manipulation techniques you can use to get anyone in the audience to help you. You could, for example, try to use the principle of "social proof". If the person does not come forward, you could ask the crowd, "What do you think, ladies and gentlemen? Should she come forward to help me?" If the crowd chants "yes" (because none of them wants to take her place), it might make the person step forward after all, because, instinctively, we humans want to be in accord with the crowd and not lose their approval.

Or, you could use the manipulation technique of "asking big and getting small". The way this works is that someone is more likely to do you a *small* favour if you asked for a *big* favour before, in contrast to asking for the *small* favour only. There are many more such techniques. However, I prefer not having to manipulate or force my volunteers if I can avoid it. I do not want them to feel bad about helping me. This brings me to the next point.

As to 2), most people will say it is obvious that your volunteers should not feel bad about helping you. But you would be surprised how often the opposite is the case. Many performers think they can sacrifice *one* in their audience for the sake of a great show for *all the others*. I do not share this attitude. I believe you should make an effort to ensure *each and everyone* who took the time to attend your show will walk away from it with the best possible feeling (I say possible, because there are some aspects you have no control over, for example men who envy you for your strength). Simply consider the repercussions. Let us assume you incorporate a family father into your show, and make him look a weakling and a fool at the same time. A weak fool, so to say. How will his wife and children, for whom he has always been a hero, feel? Or imagine you incorporate a woman into your show, and play all sorts of suggestive jokes, flirt with her, etc.? It might make her feel cheap and might make her husband furious with jealousy.

Nevertheless, many performing artists do such things routinely. How many clowns do the trick where they kiss a woman from the audience on the mouth, without her wanting it? I have also once observed a clown secretly handing a slip of paper with his telephone number to the female volunteers in his show. You can imagine how the husbands of these women felt about the clown (and the whole circus) once they found out. A clown might get away with something like this, but a strongman might not.

Thus, I always make an effort so that volunteers in my show do not have to feel bad. Of course, you will have to make your volunteer men look weaker than you, but making them look fools as well is too much. It might be a better idea to make *them* look weak, but *yourself* a fool. Then you have some kind of balance. Or, as in the earlier example, you could ask them not to *bend* a horseshoe (which they cannot, because they are "too weak"), but simply to *testify* that it is real and "impossible" to bend. When I incorporate a woman into my show, I try not to flirt with her aggressively, and if *she* does it, ignore it. Also, I try not to thematise aspects about which she might be self-conscious, such as her weight, her looks, her age, or her body. This being said, it is probably best to choose female volunteers who project an aura of self-confidence. The chances are smaller that such a woman fears losing her face, for whatever reason. Also, self-confident women are usually good sports who will enhance your show.

As mentioned, when I incorporate a child into my show, I will only use *real* volunteers. Let us assume I need a child to function as a human weight. When I sense at one point or the other that they do not want to help me any more, for whatever reason, I give them the chance to leave, saying, "You can go if you want to – no problem at all!" If they do leave, I add, "Give him a round of applause anyway, because he helped me up to this point!" Or, to increase the chances that the child will stay, you could say, "You can go if you want to – no problem at all! Of course, I would be glad if you stayed and helped me. But it is up to you." Sure, if the child leaves, your feat is ruined. But would it be better if you finished the feat without the child wanting to be part of it? I do not think so. Especially if you want to incorporate children into your show on a regular basis, it is better to signal to your audience that they do not have to fear you, children and parents likewise.

Of course, it can happen despite all these measures that a trouble-maker will stubbornly try to sabotage your show. Then, first of all, you should realize that whatever it was that made these people malevolent, was probably not their fault. This is especially true of children, for whom being malevolent can simply be an experiment, and part of a process in which they try to experience the world and learn about it. Secondly, children, as well as grown-ups, might have made bad experiences in their own lives and project this onto others. So try not to get angry, and especially do not show it yet, because this can create a bad feeling in the rest of your audience (even the benevolent viewers), and can ruin the effect of your show lastingly. As a next step, there are several possibilities:

1. Ignore the troublemaker: Many troublemakers make trouble because they want attention. It is a plausible theory that they will stop making trouble if they do not get the attention they crave. They "give up", so to say. This would be the first measure.

2. Step out of your character: If, for example, you have kept your show humorous throughout, playing jokes every now and then, and performing with a smile on your face, and then a child repeatedly tries to sabotage your show, you could try to be really serious for a minute. Step forward, look the child in the eye, and tell them, without being mean, that it needs to stop doing whatever it is that disturbs you. Otherwise you would have to speak to its parents. Sometimes this works, at least for a little while.

3. Incorporate the troublemaker into your show: Whether child or grown-up, if there is someone who repeatedly tries to disrupt your show, because they crave attention, and depriving them of this attention (i.e. ignoring them) does not help, you could try giving them the attention they crave for a minute and use them as volunteers. Maybe this will satisfy their desire for attention and silence them.

4. Make the troublemaker part of your show: If you are spontaneous and have lots of jokes at hand, you could try to play some jokes on the troublemaker and make them look a fool in front of the crowd. If you succeed, it will enhance your show by a few funny situations and will reaffirm your authority. This is obviously an aggressive method and can go painfully wrong. Use at your own risk.

Finally, know that some troublemakers have been such their whole lives and have years of experience of being a nuisance. Some are impossible to beat at their own game. In such cases there is really nothing you can do but to go on with your show and try to minimize the damage. Single persons have ruined the shows of very experienced performers.

But let me now move away again from this unpleasant topic to close this section with a different and more pleasant aspect with regard to strength demonstrations: mental strength. Above, I have already talked about the different types of performers: those who perform best when under pressure, and those whose strength performance suffers under pressure. Obviously, performing feats of strength in front of an audience equals a great amount of pressure. Image you step in front of an audience and introduce yourself as a strongman, but then fail at every feat of strength you want to demonstrate. You will make a big fool of yourself. This is exactly what people fear when they step in front of a crowd, and this is also what makes people nervous and have stage fright.

However, in the best case scenario, this fear, or pressure, can be channelled into positive energy in the form of strength. This is what works for me. I have never failed at any feat of strength I tried in front of an audience, simply because I knew (or told myself) at all times that I *must not* fail. This tells us something interesting. It demonstrates that there is a huge mental aspect about strength. One might be tempted to disregard this as esoteric, but it makes sense from a scientific perspective as well. Muscle activity is controlled on a neural level. This is also why some people express it in such a way that greater strength must not necessarily come from larger muscles, but can also result from neural adaptation, i.e. (certain types of) strength can be *learned*, rather than *built*. I do not want to claim that I understand all the science behind it, but what I do know is that I have this sort of mental strength that helps tremendously in a feat of strength whenever I step on a stage. This is an advantage I have over many other aspiring oldtime strongmen who do not perform. In a way, my shows are my training, and in them I can always utilize this mental power to do my feats of strength.

If you know yourself a little bit, you might already know which type of strength performer you are: the one who always sets personal records at competitions, or the one who is strongest in training. If you do plan to perform feats of strength in front of an audience, you will have better chances if you belong to the first type. Either way, performing feats of strength in front of an audience will help you to build and hone this mental strength. Eventually, if you try hard enough, you might manage to become habituated to developing a similar attitude in your training, or at least to retrieve this additional mental strength for personal record attempts.

20. Epilogue: My addendum to Arthur Saxon's definition of a strong man

For whatever reason you picked up this book, whether you were only interested in my training techniques, whether you want to try oldtime strongman training to build old-fashioned all-round strength, or whether you have plans to step on a stage and perform oldtime strongman feats yourself, I hope my ideas will be of service. I have tried to cover lots of different aspects in this book. Some further aspects I could not cover for reasons of space, and maybe I also talked about some things you were not interested in. Either way, I hope you will pardon my selection.

I also hope you did not expect to read of any "secrets" – perhaps any mysterious and forgotten (East-) German training techniques, which were lost and which I recovered, and which will enable you to build strength and muscle mass quickly, without effort. I could not disclose these secrets, simply because there are none – at least none that I know of. The only "secrets" the German strongmen of the golden era had were their Prussian virtues: determination, discipline, industriousness, toughness, fortitude, order, straightness, etc. (there are some others that I am not so fond of).

I needed no other "secrets" to achieve the results I did. I always tell those people who envy me for my strength and muscles that I started lifting weights at age thirteen (and have never stopped since then). As a young man, when my fellow classmates drank and partied at the weekends, I drank a glass of milk and went to bed early. The next morning, I got up early, went swimming for an hour, got home, breakfasted, and lifted weights, while they were still snoring in their beds. I had a lot less fun than they, but I had training results. It was a simple trade.

In any case, whatever you make of the information in this book, I would be happy if you used it as a means to a good end – not for purely narcissistic, arrogant, or egotistical endeavours. Oldtime strongman training is, by definition, an anachronism, a nostalgic step backwards. With this book, I do not want to say that one should deny all the advancements humanity has made since the golden age of the strongmen. However, I believe that, at least in some respects, the world could become a better place if we went back in time, and recalled past attitudes, technologies, and ways of living, which were better for the human body and mind, because they were simpler, and better for our world, because they were more sustainable.

I want to close this book by recalling Arthur Saxon's definition of strength from 1906 once more:

"Genuine strength should include not only momentary strength, as proved by the ability to lift a heavy weight once, but also the far more valuable kind of strength known as strength for endurance. This means the ability, if you are a cyclist, to jump on your machine and ride 100 miles at any time without undue fatigue; if a wrestler, to wrestle a hard bout for half an hour with a good man without a rest, yet without becoming exhausted and reaching the limit of your strength.

Apart from sports, enduring strength means that the business man shall stand, without a break-down, business cares and worries, that he shall be capable, when necessary, of working morning, afternoon and night with unflagging energy, holding tightly in his grasp he reins of business, retaining all the while a clear mind and untiring energy, both of body and brain. The man who can miss a night's rest or miss a meal or two without showing any ill effect or without losing any physical power, is better entitled to be considered a strong man than the man who is only apparently strong, being possessed of momentary strength, which is, after all, a muscle test pure and simple. In the latter case, where a man raises, once only, a heavy weight, all that he proves himself to possess is muscular control and great contractile power, but this does not guarantee sound internal organs, nor does it prove that a man would come out well in an endurance test." (Saxon 23-24)

To this, I would like to add:

"A strong man is to me also someone with a strong character. Someone who utilizes his strength for the good of mankind, to help other (weaker) people, to protect others, to be a positive role model, to be an inspiration, and to promote a healthy and sustainable lifestyle, to the best of his knowledge and abilities."

List of illustrations

Figure 1.1 *Friedrich August "der Starke" I. von Sachsen.*
Source: Wikimedia Commons. Public domain.

Figure 1.2 *Milo Barus.*
Postcard, c. 1960.

Figure 4.1 *Acrobat and highwire artist Walter Moshammer from Austria.*
Courtesy of Walter Moshammer.

Figure 5.1 *Sportsmen in ancient Greece.*
Edward Norman Gardiner (1864-1930), *Greek Athletic Sports and Festivals* (1910). Source: Flickr. No known restrictions.

Figure 5.2 *Greek wrestlers in antiquity.*
Edward Norman Gardiner (1864-1930), *Greek Athletic Sports and Festivals* (1910). Source: Flickr. No known restrictions.

Figure 5.3 *Palaeolithic activities.*
Wiktor Michailowitsch Wasnezow (1848-1926), "Stone Age". Source: Wikimedia Commons. Public domain in its country of origin and other countries and areas where the copyright term is the author's life plus 80 years or fewer. Photographic reproduction.

Figure 6.1 *Getting ready for nail driving.*

Figure 7.1 *Pull-ups on slings of rope.*

Figure 8.1 *Atlas stone with additional weight.*

Figure 9.1 *Natural stonelifting.*
Based on photograph by Bert Walser.

Figure 9.2 *Shouldering the Inver Stone.*

Figure 9.3 *Lifting the Dinnie Stones.*

Figure 9.4 *With a harness, a strong man can theoretically lift a horse.*
Circus strongman in Brisbane, Australia (1903). Source: Flickr. No known restrictions.

Figure 9.5 *My self-made lifting platform (here used for a teeth lift).*

Figure 9.6 *Eighteenth-century engraving of British strongman Thomas Topham performing a harness lift. One of the historical models on which I based my lifting platform.*
C. Leigh, after William Henry Toms, "Thomas Topham, lifting 1836 lbs." (1741). Source: Wellcome Library, London. Copyrighted work available under Creative Commons Attribution only licence CC BY 4.0.

Figure 9.7 *Nail bending with the underhand technique.*
Based on photograph by Paul Gruber.

Figure 9.8 *John Grün.*
Courtesy of Georges Christen.

Figure 9.9 *Nail bending with the overhand technique.*

Figure 9.10 *Horseshoe bending.*
Based on photograph by Dennis Jarczyk.

Figure 9.11 *A horseshoe bent to 180 degrees.*

Figure 9.12 *An Inch-style dumbbell lifted overhead.*

Figure 9.13 *Setting a hand gripper (above) and closing a hand gripper (below).*
Based on photograph by Bert Walser.

Figure 9.14 *My leather mouthpiece.*

Figure 9.15 *Mouthpieces of artificial material.*

Figure 9.16 *The famous strongman Siegmund Breitbart getting ready for a towing feat. The hefty chains and mouthpiece suggest a heavy load.*
"Siegmund 'Zishe' Breitbart, performer/strongman who used his teeth to pull a wagon with 50 persons on board through the streets of Washington, D.C., 11/27/23." Source: Library of Congress, Prints & Photographs Division, LC-DIG-npcc-09986 (digital file from original). No known restrictions.

Figure 9.17 *Strongman Chris "Hairculese" Rider with a one-cent coin he has bent.*
Courtesy of Chris Rider.

Figure 9.18 *Strongman Rainer Schröder bending a horseshoe with his teeth.*
Courtesy of Rainer Schröder.

Figure 9.19 *Strongman Georges Christen bending three nails with his teeth.*
Source: Georges Christen Archive. Courtesy of Georges Christen.

Figure 9.20 *The chair balancing feat.*
Based on photograph by Manfred Storf.

Figure 9.21 *The table supporting feat.*
Based on photograph by Friedrich Klawiter.

Figure 9.22 *The overhead catch.*

Figure 9.23 *A sideward flip with two kettlebells.*
Based on photograph by Friedrich Klawiter.

Figure 9.24 *Strongman Mighty Mike from Canada.*
Courtesy of Mike Johns.

Figure 12.1 *Levering exercise with a sledgehammer.*

Figure 13.1 *A stereotypical illustration of an oldtime strongman.*

Figure 13.2 *The wiry type: Joseph "The Mighty Atom" Greenstein.*
Source: Flickr. Licensed under the terms of the United States Government Work.

Figure 13.3 *The brawny type: George Hackenschmidt.*
Autograph card, c. 1905. Source: Wikimedia Commons. Public domain.

Figure 13.4 *The overweight type: Emil Naucke.*
"Mr E. Naucke, weighing 410 lbs." Source: Wellcome Library, London. Copyrighted work available under Creative Commons Attribution licence CC BY 4.0. No changes made.

Figure 13.5 *The great Louis Cyr.*
Source: Wikimedia Commons. Public domain.

Figure 15.1 *HRH Charles, Prince of Wales.*
"Charles, Prince of Wales, in a meeting with José Luis Rodríguez Zapatero" (31 March 2011). Source: Wikimedia Commons. Copyright holder: Ministry of the Presidency, Government of Spain.

Figure 18.1 *Adrian Peter Schmidt.*
    Source: Wikimedia Commons. Public domain.

Figure 19.1 *Performing in the circus.*

Sources

Bonini, Gherardo, Mark Kodya, and Joe Roark. "Was Hermann Goerner Truly Mighty?" *Iron Game History* 9.4 (2007): 21-32.

Brookfield, John. "The Slaying of Goliath: Bending a Red Nail." *MILO: A Journal for Serious Strength Athletes* 11.4 (2004): 44-46.

Chandler, Steve. *Time Warrior: How to Defeat Procrastination, People-Pleasing, Over-Commitment, Broken Promises and Chaos.* Anna Maria: Maurice Bassett, 2011.

Cordain, Loren. *The Paleo-Diet.* Hoboken, NJ: Wiley, 2002.

Crowther, Nigel B. *Athletika: Studies on the Olympic Games and Greek Athletics.* Hildesheim: Weidmann, 2004.

Crowther, Nigel B., and Monika Frass. „Bodyb(u)ilder im Altertum - verehrt oder verachtet?" *Körper im Kopf: Antike Diskurse zum Körper.* Ed. P. Mauritsch. Graz: Leykam, 2010. 143-167.

Engels, Friedrich. *Der Ursprung der Familie, des Privateigentums und des Staats.* Hottingen-Zürich: Schweizer. genoss. Buchdr., 1884.

Franklin, Benjamin. *The Autobiography & Other Writings by Benjamin Franklin.* Ed. Peter Shaw. New York et al.: Bantam, 1982.

Gröning, Flora. "Kiefer und Zähne der am besten erforschten fossilen Menschenform: Neanderthalers starkes Gebiss." *Dental Magazin* 3 (2006): 116-119.

Groth, Lothar. *Die starken Männer: Eine Geschichte der Kraftakrobatik.* Berlin: Henschelverlag, 1987.

Jeck, Steve, and Peter Martin. *Of Stones and Strength.* Nevada: IronMind, 1996.

Lechler, Tobias. *Die Ernährung als Einflussfaktor auf die Evolution des Menschen.* Doctoral thesis. University of Hanover, 2001.

Lee, Richard B. *The Cambridge Encyclopedia of Hunters and Gatherers.* Cambridge: Cambridge University Press, 1999.

London, Jack. *The Sea-Wolf.* New York: Grosset, 1938.

MacMahon, Charles. *Feats of Strength and Dexterity.* 1927. Reprint ed. Farmington: Hinbern, 2000.

McDougall, Christopher. *Born to Run: Ein vergessenes Volk und das Geheimnis der besten und glücklichsten Läufer der Welt.* Trans. Werner Roller. München: Blessing, 2010.

McKay, Brett, and Kate McKay. "Odd Exercises for Physical Vigor: An Oldtime Strongman's 15-Minute Morning Routine." *The Art of Manliness.* 15 May 2014.
<https://www.artofmanliness.com/articles/odd-exercises-for-physical-vigor-an-oldtime-strongmans-15-minute-morning-routine/>

McKee, Robert. *Story: Substance, Structure, Style, and the Principles of Screenwriting.* New York: HarperCollins, 1997.

Moser, Thorsten. *Hans Steyrer: Bayerischer Herkules.* Norderstedt: Books on Demand, 2011.

Mueller, Edgar. *Goerner the Mighty.* 1951. N.p.: O'Faolain Patriot, 2012.

Price, Weston A. *Nutrition and Physical Degeneration: A Comparison of Primitive and Modern Diets and their Effects, etc.* New York: Hoeber, 1939.

Pyle, Howard. *Robin Hood.* Bindlach: Loewe, n.d.

Rosseau, Jean-Jacques. *Abhandlung über den Ursprung und die Grundlagen der Ungleichheit unter den Menschen.* 1755. Ed. and trans. Philipp Rippel. Stuttgart: Reclam, 1998.

Saxon, Arthur. *The Development of Physical Power.* 1906. N.p.: O'Faolain Patriot, 2011.

Schmidt, Adrian Peter. *Illustrated Hints for Health and Strength for Busy People.* New Yok: published by the author, 1901.

Spindler, Robert, and Tommy Heslep. *Grip Strength: How to Close Heavy Duty Hand Grippers, Lift Thick Bar Weights and Pinch Grip just about anything.* Innsbruck: published by the author, 2013.

Veblen, Thorstein. *The Theory of the Leisure Class: An Economic Study of Institutions.* New York: Viking, 1945.

Weiler, Ingomar. *Der Sport bei den Völkern der Alten Welt.* Darmstadt: Wissenschaftliche Buchgesellschaft, 1981.

Zarnowski, Frank. "The Amazing Donald Dinnie: The Nineteenth Century's Greatest Athlete." *Iron Game History* 5.1 (1998): 3-11.

Zeimet, Frank. *John Grün: Muskelkraft und Welterfolg. Mit einem Zusatz über George Christen.* Luxemburger Biographien 3. Luxemburg: Sankt-Paulus-Druckerei, 1989.

DID YOU LIKE THIS BOOK?

Whether yes or no, you can do me a great favour:

Write me a short mail, saying what you liked or did not like about the book at

robert.spindler@gmail.com

Just give me a short feedback.

I am trying to improve my products constantly, to help my readers become strong and stay healthy the best way possible.

Thank you.

ALSO AVAILABLE:

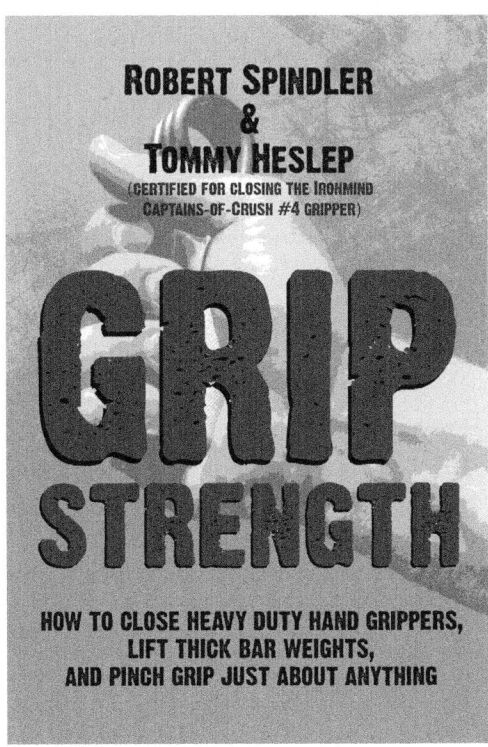

ROBERT SPINDLER
&
TOMMY HESLEP
(CERTIFIED FOR CLOSING THE IRONMIND
CAPTAINS-OF-CRUSH #4 GRIPPER)

GRIP
STRENGTH

HOW TO CLOSE HEAVY DUTY HAND GRIPPERS,
LIFT THICK BAR WEIGHTS,
AND PINCH GRIP JUST ABOUT ANYTHING

Printed in Great Britain
by Amazon

62508673R00139